W9-AVL-677

DENTAL
RADIOGRAPHIC
DIAGNOSIS

SECOND EDITION

DENTAL RADIOGRAPHIC DIAGNOSIS

SECOND EDITION

KAVAS H. THUNTHY, B.D.S. M.S., M.ED.

Board Certified,
American Board of Oral and Maxillofacial Radiology
Professor, Oral and Maxillofacial Radiology
Department of Oral Diagnosis, Medicine and Radiology

Louisiana State University
School of Dentistry
New Orleans, Louisiana, U.S.A.

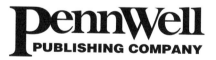

DENTAL ECONOMICS

PennWell Publishing Company
Tulsa, Oklahoma

This book is dedicated to
Students of Dentistry
For their Dreams and Sacrifices

Copyright © 1997 by
PennWell Publishing Company
1421 South Sheridan/P.O. Box 1260
Tulsa, Oklahoma 74101

Thunthy, Kavas H.
    Dental radiographic diagnosis/b Kavas H. Thunthy.—2nd ed.
        p.   cm.
    Includes index.
    ISBN 0-87814-706-3
    1. Teeth—Radiography. 2. Mouth—Radiography. I. Title.
    [DNLM: 1. Radiography, Dental—atlases 2. Tooth Diseases—atlases. 3. Mouth Diseases—atlases. 4.
Jaw Diseases—atlases. WN 17 T535d 1997]
    RK309.T495 1997
    617.6'07572—dc21
    DNLM/DLC
    for Library of Congress   96-47747
                                                                                          CIP

Printed in the United States of America

1 2 3 4 5 01 00 99 98 97

PREFACE

The experience gained from writing the first edition has enabled me to rework and modify the book for the second edition. The primary theme of the book remains unchanged: to provide students and dental clinicians with basic information to function in clinical situations using conventional radiographs. The material is presented in a concise illustrative format that can readily be absorbed by students. It is not intended for advanced knowledge of the subject matter nor is it intended to include advanced imaging modalities. There are no illustrations dealing with tomography, computed tomography, and magnetic resonance imaging; I have intentionally excluded them. After studying the book the reader will be able to confidently interpret images on conventional radiographs and correlate them to normal and disease processes. In summation, the simplified format makes the book easy for learning.

For practical reasons, every book has limits on information to be included. Therefore, I have omitted the following five chapters from the second edition because adequate coverage was not possible on a few pages: "Sialograms," "Evaluation of Laboratory Chemistries," "Edosseous Implants," "Jaw Fractures," and "Temporomandibular Joint." I have combined the chapters on "Developmental Disturbances" and "Endocrine and Other Systemic Disorders" into "Genetic and Metabolic Diseases". I have made no significant change to the chapters on normal anatomy, but I have expanded descriptive texts in most of the chapters. With the elimination of redundant illustrations, the second edition contains about 160 fewer illustrations than the first edition. I have streamlined the book without sacrificing quality, so that it will be more affordable for students.

ACKNOWLEDGMENTS

I dedicate this book to students of dentistry who challenge me to succeed as an educator and who give me great joy and fulfillment in my work.

For this second edition, I would like to acknowledge the following individuals for their valued assistance: Maureen Raymond, Fern Hoffman, and Lynn Christian for their secretarial services, Bob Raben for his photographic services, and Michael Higgins for his editorial services.

I would like to thank Dr. Eric Hovland, Dean of the Louisiana State University School of Dentistry, for the use of dental school personnel and facilities.

I also appreciate the suggestions and cooperation of the staff of PennWell Publishing Company, especially Mr. Kirk Bjornsgaard, dental editor.

CONTENTS

CHAPTER 1
Normal Radiographic Anatomy • 1
A. Maxillary anatomic landmarks • 1
B. Mandibular anatomic landmarks • 21
C. Restorative materials • 33

CHAPTER 2
Panoramic Anatomy • 41

CHAPTER 3
Patient Positioning Errors in Panoramic Radiography • 51

CHAPTER 4
Extraoral and Occlusal Anatomic Landmarks • 57

CHAPTER 5
Dental Caries • 75

CHAPTER 6
Periodontal Disease • 91

CHAPTER 7
Apical Lesions • 103

CHAPTER 8
Technique Errors and Artifacts • 137

CHAPTER 9
Foreign Bodies in and about the Jaws • *155*

CHAPTER 10
Dental Anomalies • *169*

CHAPTER 11
Soft Tissue Calcifications • *217*

CHAPTER 12
Cysts of the Jaws • *231*

CHAPTER 13
Osteomyelitis • *267*

CHAPTER 14
Odontogenic Benign Tumors of the Jaws • *279*

CHAPTER 15
Nonodontogenic Benign Tumors of the Jaws • *305*

CHAPTER 16
Malignant Tumors of the Jaws • *327*

CHAPTER 17
Maxillary Sinus * *343*

CHAPTER 18
Genetic and Metabolic Diseases • *365*

CHAPTER 19
Differential Diagnosis of Common Lesions • *407*

INDEX • *415*

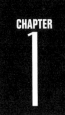

NORMAL RADIOGRAPHIC ANATOMY

INTRAORAL LANDMARKS

MAXILLARY ANATOMIC LANDMARKS

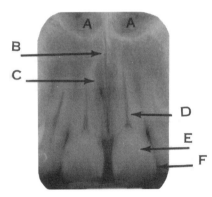

Figure 1–1
- A—Nasal fossae (nasal cavities)
- B—Median palatine suture (intermaxillary suture)
- C—Incisive foramen (anterior palatine foramen)
- D—Root canal
- E—Dentin
- F—Enamel

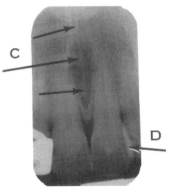

Figure 1–2
- C—Median palatine suture (intermaxillary suture)
- D—Overlapping of teeth

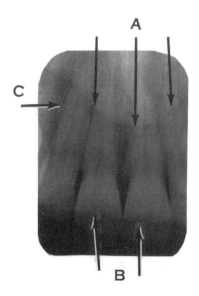

Figure 1–3
A—Soft tissue of nose
B—Upper lip line (border of a
heavy upper lip)
C—Lamina dura (radiopaque line)
and periodontal ligament space
(radiolucent line) surrounding
the tooth root

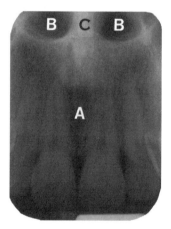

Figure 1–4
A—Incisive foramen (anterior
palatine foramen)
B—Nasal fossae (nasal cavities)
C—Nasal septum

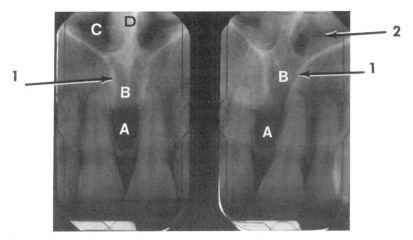

Figure 1–5
> A—Incisive foramen
> B—Incisive canal (nasopalatine canal, anterior palatine canal)
> C—Nasal fossa (nasal cavity)
> D—Nasal septum covered on each side by nasal mucosa
> 1—Walls of the incisive canal
> 2—Inferior nasal meatus

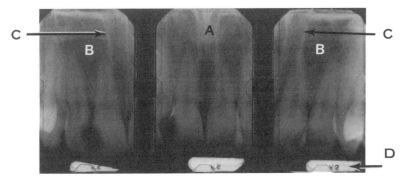

Figure 1–6
> A—Incisive canal (nasopalatine canal)
> B—Lateral fossa (thin bone)
> C—Walls of the incisive canal
> D—Metal x–ray instrument

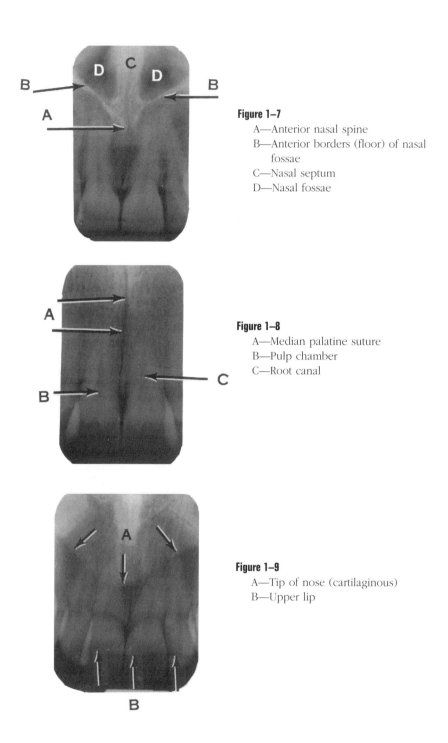

Figure 1–7
    A—Anterior nasal spine
    B—Anterior borders (floor) of nasal
        fossae
    C—Nasal septum
    D—Nasal fossae

Figure 1–8
    A—Median palatine suture
    B—Pulp chamber
    C—Root canal

Figure 1–9
    A—Tip of nose (cartilaginous)
    B—Upper lip

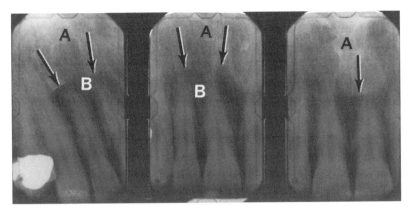

Figure 1–10
  A—Soft tissue of nose (arrows)
  B—Lateral fossa (due to thinness of bone)

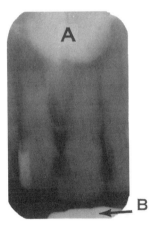

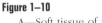

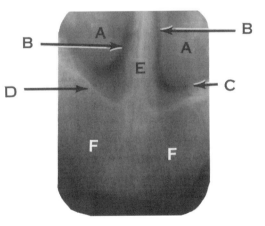

Figure 1–11
  A—Palatal torus (torus palatinus)
  B—X–ray instrument

Figure 1–12
  A—Inferior nasal conchae (turbinate bones)
  B—Common nasal meatus
  C—Inferior nasal meatus
  D—Anterior border (floor) of nasal fossa
  E—Nasal septum
  F—Trabeculae in the maxillary bone.
    Compare this trabecular pattern with that in the mandibular bone

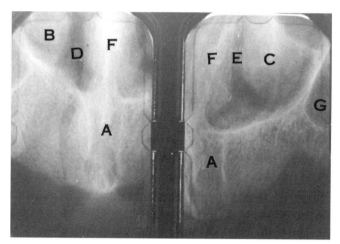

Figure 1–13

Radiographs mounted with film bumps facing the reader

A—Incisive canal

B—Patient's right inferior nasal concha

C—Patient's left inferior nasal concha

D—Patient's right common nasal meatus

E—Patient's left common nasal meatus

F—Nasal septum

G—Patient's left maxillary sinus

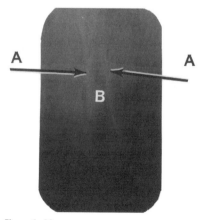

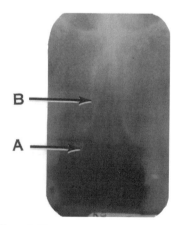

Figure 1–14

Edentulous maxilla–midline region

A—Walls of the incisive canal

B—Incisive canal (nasopalatine canal)

Figure 1–15

A—Soft tissue (gingiva)

B—Wall of the nasopalatine canal

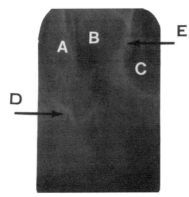

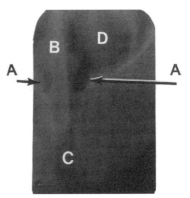

Figure 1–16
- A—Nasal septum
- B—Patient's left nasal fossa (containing inferior nasal concha)
- C—Maxillary sinus (of patient's left side when film bump faces the reader)
- D—Anterior nasal spine
- E—Anterior wall of the maxillary sinus

Figure 1–17
- A—Superior foramina of the incisive canal
- B—Nasal septum
- C—Incisive canal connecting the incisive foramen to the superior foramina of the incisive canal
- D—Nasal fossa (of patient's left side when film bump faces the reader)

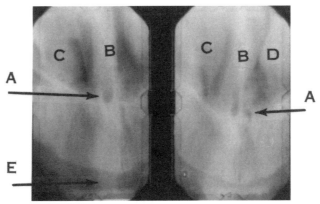

Figure 1–18
- A—Superior foramina of the incisive canal
- B—Nasal septum (bony) covered on each side by nasal mucosa
- C—Inferior nasal concha (of patient's right side when film bump faces the reader)
- D—Inferior nasal concha (of patient's left side when film bump faces the reader)
- E—Cartilaginous septum of nose

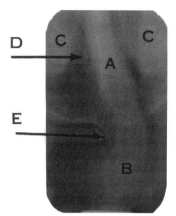

Figure 1–19
A—Nasal septum (bony)
B—Cartilaginous septum of nose
C—Inferior nasal conchae
D—Common nasal meatus
E—Anterior nasal spine

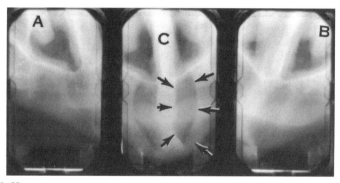

Figure 1–20
Arrows–External naris of the patient's left side (plural.nares)

A—Inferior nasal concha (of patient's right side when film bump faces the reader)

B—Inferior nasal concha (of patient's left side when film bump faces the reader)

C—Nasal septum (bony) The three arrows directly below "C" are superimposed on the cartilaginous nasal septum. The other three arrows on the side are superimposed on the left ala of the nose

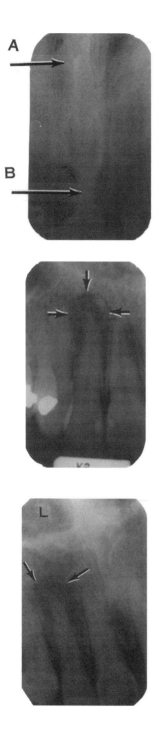

Figure 1–21
> A—Bony nasal septum
> B—Cartilaginous nasal septum

Figure 1–22
> Arrows—Lateral fossa (radiolucent image produced by the thinness of bone)
>
> The lateral fossa could be misdiagnosed as an apical lesion and should, therefore, be compared with the contralateral side. When in doubt, pulp vitality test should be performed to differentiate a lateral fossa from an inflammatory apical lesion.

Figure 1–23
> Arrows—Lateral fossa (radiolucent image produced by the thinness of bone)
>
> The lateral fossa could be misdiagnosed as an apical lesion
>
> L—Patient's right nasal fossa (when film bump faces the reader)

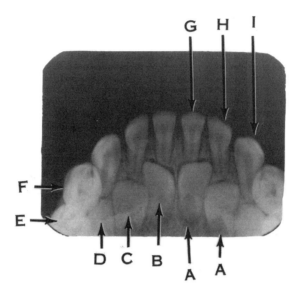

Figure 1–24
A—Dental papillae of unerupted permanent central and lateral incisors
B—Unerupted permanent central incisor (mandibular)
C—Unerupted permanent lateral incisor
D—Unerupted permanent canine
E—Right deciduous second molar
F—Right deciduous first molar
G—Left deciduous central incisor
H—Left deciduous lateral incisor
I—Left deciduous canine

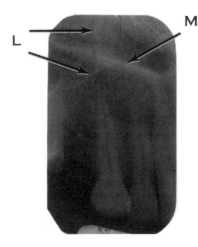

Figure 1–25
L—Anterior wall of maxillary sinus
M—Anterior border (floor) of nasal fossa

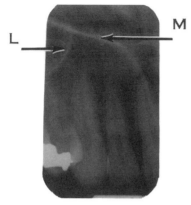

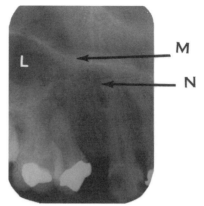

Figure 1–26

L—Anterior wall of maxillary sinus
M—Anterior border (floor) of nasal
   fossa

Figure 1–27

L—Maxillary sinus (antrum)
M—Anterior border (floor) of nasal
   fossa
N—Nutrient canal leading to a
   nutrient foramen

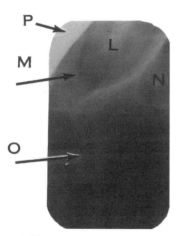

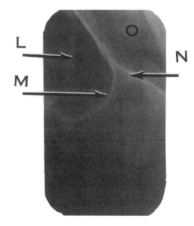

Figure 1–28

L—Inferior nasal concha (turbinate)
M—Inferior nasal meatus
N—Maxillary sinus (of patient's left
   side when film bump faces the
   reader)
O—Ala of nose (soft tissue)
P—Slight cone cut (technique error)

Figure 1–29

L—Septum in maxillary sinus
M—Anterior wall of right maxillary
   sinus
N—Anterior border (floor) of nasal
   fossa
O—Patient's right nasal fossa

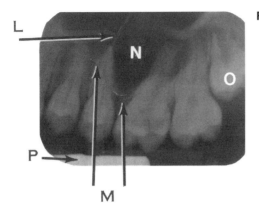

Figure 1–30

L—Septum in maxillary sinus

M—Floor of maxillary sinus

N—Maxillary sinus (antrum)

O—Unerupted third molar

P—X–ray dental instrument (metal rod)

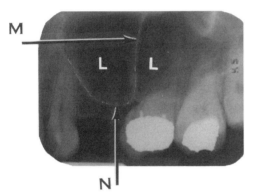

Figure 1–31

L—Maxillary sinus (antrum)

M—Septum in maxillary sinus

N—Floor of maxillary sinus

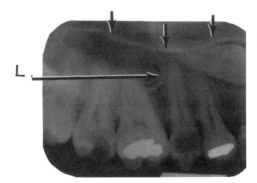

Figure 1–32

Arrows—Floor of nasal fossa (junction of the lateral wall and floor of nasal fossa)

L—Anterior wall of maxillary sinus

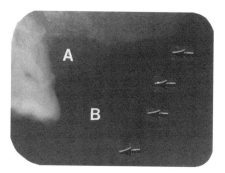

Figure 1–33

Arrows—Nasolabial fold

A—Gingiva
B—Cheek

The radiograph is of the patient's right side when the film bump faces the reader

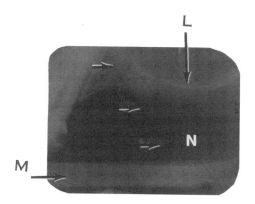

Figure 1–34

Arrows—Nasolabial fold

L—Floor of maxillary sinus
M—Plastic x–ray
    instrument
    (Snap.A.Ray®)
N—Cheek

The radiograph is of the patient's left side when the film bump faces the reader

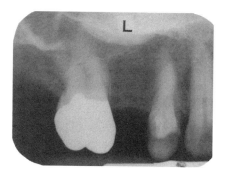

Figure 1–35
L—Torus palatinus

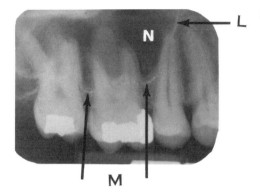

Figure 1–36

L—Anterior wall of maxillary sinus

M—Floor of the maxillary sinus

N—Maxillary sinus (antrum)

Notice that the roots of the molars project into the sinus

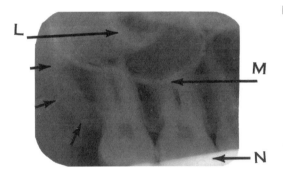

Figure 1–37

Small arrows— Maxillary tuberosity

L—Zygomatic process of maxilla (U–shaped)

M—Floor of maxillary sinus

N—Dental instrument (hemostat) superimposed on the crowns of teeth

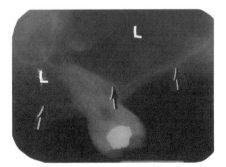

Figure 1–38

L—Maxillary sinus

Arrows—Floor of maxillary sinus

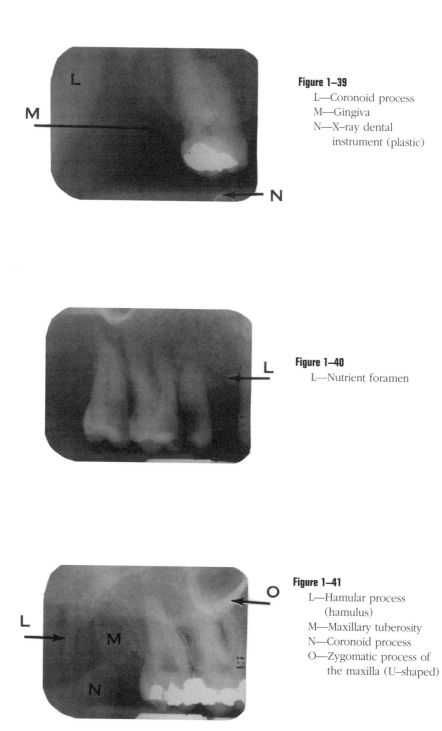

Figure 1–39
 L—Coronoid process
 M—Gingiva
 N—X–ray dental
  instrument (plastic)

Figure 1–40
 L—Nutrient foramen

Figure 1–41
 L—Hamular process
  (hamulus)
 M—Maxillary tuberosity
 N—Coronoid process
 O—Zygomatic process of
  the maxilla (U–shaped)

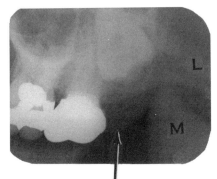

Figure 1–42
    L—Zygomatic arch
    M—Coronoid process
    N—Gingiva

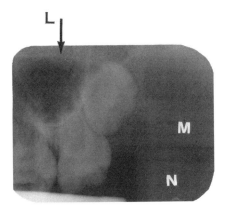

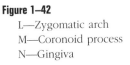

Figure 1–43
    L—Floor of the nasal
        cavity
    M—Zygomatic arch
    N—Coronoid process

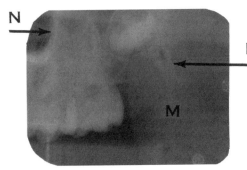

Figure 1–44
    L—Pterygoid plates
    M—Coronoid process
    N—Zygomatic process of
        the maxilla (U–shaped)

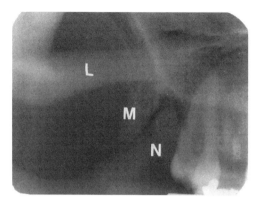

Figure 1–45

L— Zygomatic arch

M—Pterygoid plates

N—Coronoid process

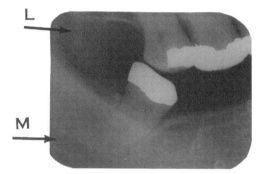

Figure 1–46

Bite-wing radiograph

L—Hamular process

M—Mandibular canal

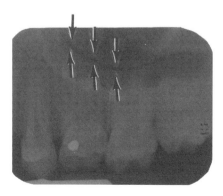

Figure 1–47

Arrows—Vascular canal (or groove) in the lateral wall of maxillary sinus.

Canal (or groove) for the posterior superior alveolar artery

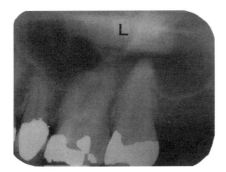

Figure 1–48
L—Torus palatinus

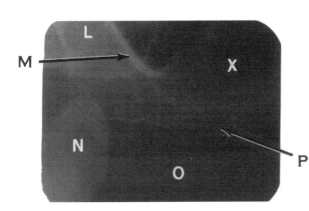

Figure 1–49
The radiograph is of the patient's right side when film bump faces the reader

L—Zygoma (malar bone)
M—Zygomatic process of maxilla (U–shaped)
N—Coronoid process
O—X–ray dental instrument (plastic)
P—Alveolar ridge
X—Maxillary sinus

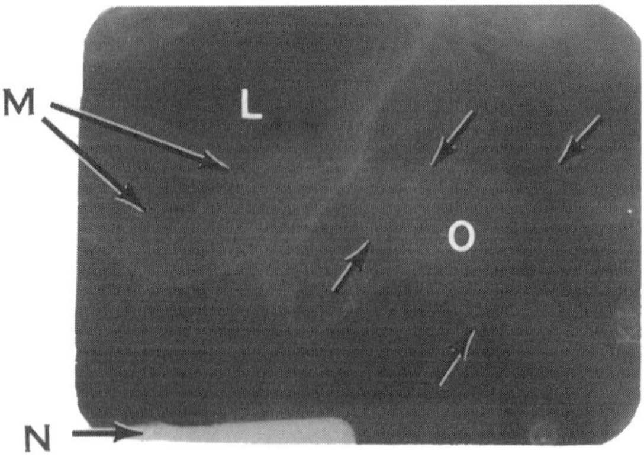

Figure 1–50
The radiograph is of the patient's left side when film bump faces the reader

L—Maxillary sinus (antrum)
M—Thickened mucosal lining of sinus
N—X–ray dental instrument (metal rod)
O and surrounded by four arrows—Coronoid process

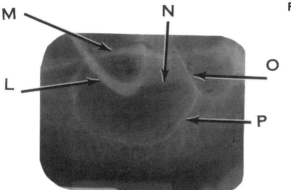

Figure 1–51

The radiograph is of the patient's left side when film bump faces the reader

L—Zygomatic process of the maxilla (U–shaped)
M—Floor of the nasal fossa (junction of lateral wall and floor of nasal fossa)
N—Inferior border of the zygoma
O—Septum in maxillary sinus
P—Floor of maxillary sinus

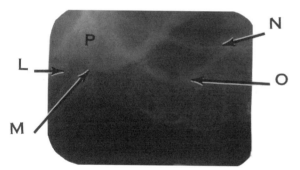

Figure 1–52

The radiograph is of the patient's right side when film bump faces the reader

L—Maxillary tuberosity
M—Inferior border of zygoma
N—Floor of nasal cavity
O—Floor of maxillary sinus
P—Zygoma (malar bone)

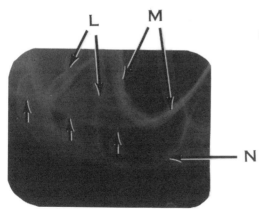

Figure 1–53

The radiograph is of the patient's right side when film bump faces the reader
Small arrows–inferior border of zygoma

L—Septa in maxillary sinus
M—Zygomatic process of maxilla (U–shaped)
N—Floor of maxillary sinus (near the alveolar ridge surface)

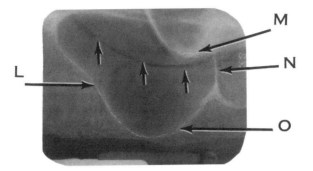

Figure 1–54

The radiograph is of the patient's left side when film bump faces the reader

Small arrows—Vascular canal (or groove) in lateral wall of maxillary sinus. Canal (or groove) for the posterior superior alveolar artery

L—Anterior wall of maxillary sinus
M—Zygomatic process of maxilla
N—Septum in maxillary sinus
O—Floor of maxillary sinus

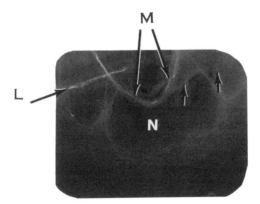

Figure 1–55

The radiograph is of the patient's left side when film bump faces the reader
Small arrows–inferior border of zygoma

L—Floor of nasal fossa
M—Zygomatic process of the maxilla (U–shaped)
N—Maxillary sinus

MANDIBULAR ANATOMIC LANDMARKS

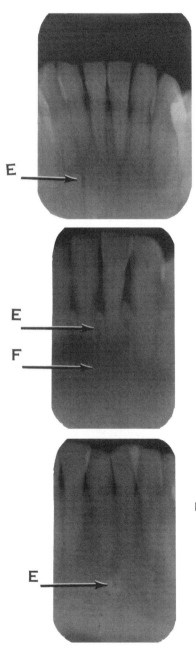

Figure 1–56
E—Nutrient canals

Figure 1–57
E—Nutrient foramen
F—Nutrient canal

Figure 1–58
E—Genial tubercles (circular
    radiopacity) surrounding lingual
    foramen (radiolucent dot)

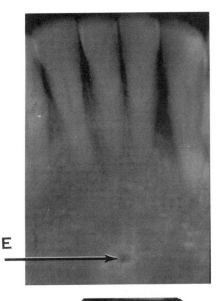

Figure 1–59
E—Genial tubercles (circular radiopacity) surrounding lingual foramen (radiolucent dot)

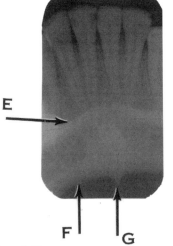

Figure 1–60
E—Mental ridge
F—Inferior border of mandible
G—Genial tubercles appear to arise from the lower border of the mandible because of excessive negative angulation of the x–ray beam

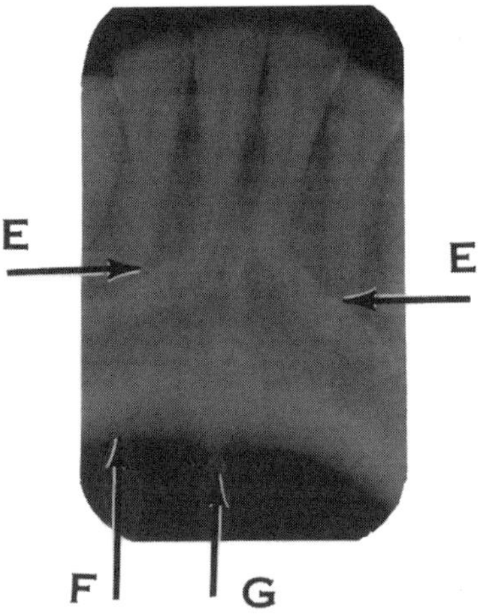

Figure 1–61
E—Mental ridges
F—Inferior border of mandible
G—Genial tubercles.
Overangulation of the x–ray beam produced the illusion of the genial tubercles arising from the inferior border of the mandible.

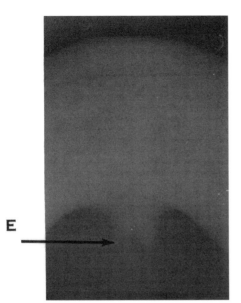

Figure 1–62
 E—Genial tubercles (as
  seen on an occlusal
  film) protrude lingually

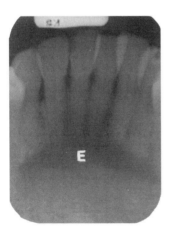

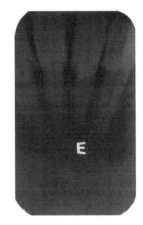

Figure 1–63
 E—Mental fossa (depression in
  bone)

The mental fossa could be
misdiagnosed as an apical lesion

Figure 1–64
 E—Mental fossa (depression in
  bone)

The mental fossa could be
misdiagnosed as an apical lesion

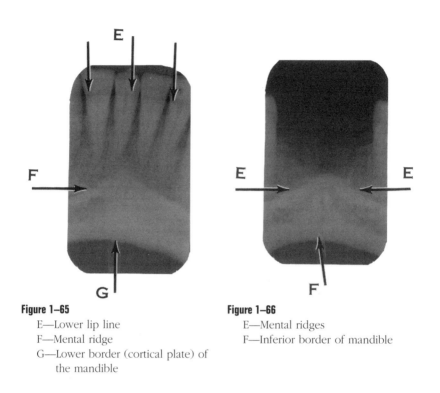

Figure 1–65
E—Lower lip line
F—Mental ridge
G—Lower border (cortical plate) of
the mandible

Figure 1–66
E—Mental ridges
F—Inferior border of mandible

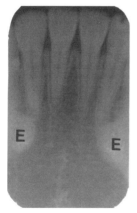

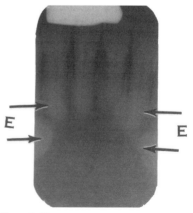

Figure 1–67
E—Mandibular tori

Figure 1–68
E—Mandibular tori

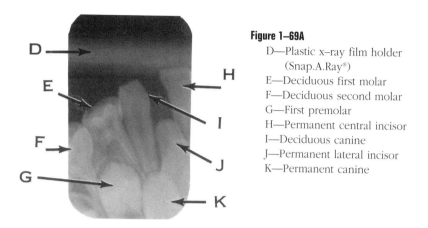

Figure 1–69A

D—Plastic x–ray film holder (Snap.A.Ray®)
E—Deciduous first molar
F—Deciduous second molar
G—First premolar
H—Permanent central incisor
I—Deciduous canine
J—Permanent lateral incisor
K—Permanent canine

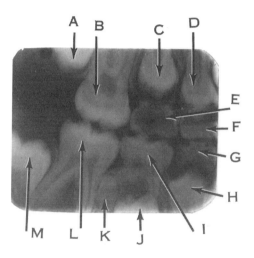

Figure 1–69B

Bite–wing radiograph of patient's right side

A—Unerupted maxillary second permanent molar
B—Maxillary first permanent molar
C—Unerupted maxillary second premolar
D—Unerupted maxillary first premolar
E—Maxillary second deciduous molar
F—Maxillary first deciduous molar
G—Mandibular first deciduous molar

H—Unerupted mandibular first premolar
I—Mandibular second deciduous molar
J—Unerupted mandibular second premolar
K—Supernumerary tooth (unerupted)
L—Mandibular permanent first molar
M—Unerupted mandibular permanent second molar

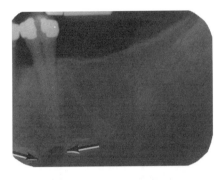

Figure 1–70
Mental foramen

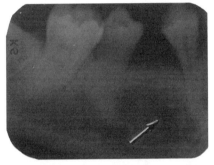

Figure 1–71
Mental foramen

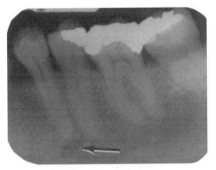

Figure 1–72
Mental foramen. May be
mistaken as an apical lesion

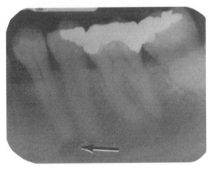

Figure 1–73A
Mental foramen image
superimposed on the apex of the
first premolar because of
overangulation of the x–ray beam

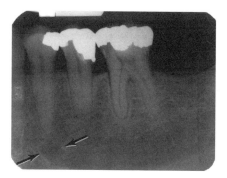

Figure 1–73B

Mental foramen. Correct x–ray beam angulation is used. The foramen is no longer superimposed on the root apex. This change in position of the radiolucency with changes in x–ray beam angulation differentiates an anatomy from an apical lesion.

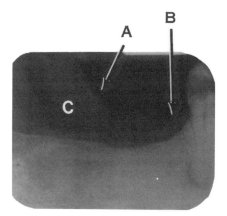

Figure 1–74

A—Nasolabial fold
B—Gingiva
C—Cheek

The radiograph is of the patient's right side when film bump faces the reader

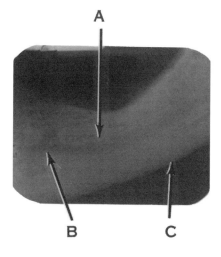

Figure 1–75

A—Mandibular canal
B—Mental foramen
C—Inferior border of mandible (cortical bone)

The radiograph is of the patient's left side when film bump faces the reader

27

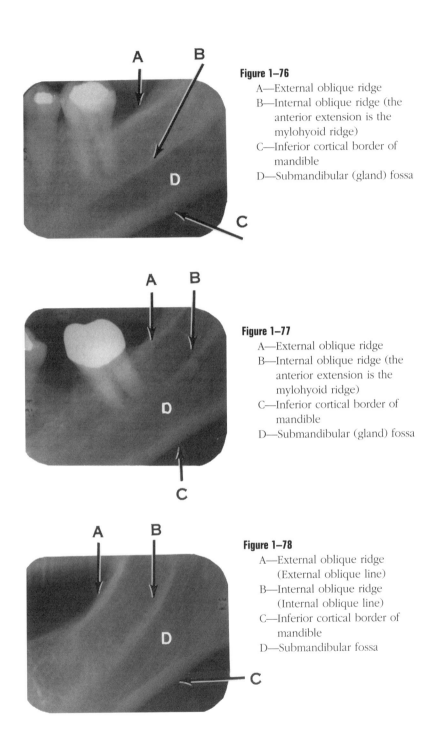

Figure 1–76
A—External oblique ridge
B—Internal oblique ridge (the anterior extension is the mylohyoid ridge)
C—Inferior cortical border of mandible
D—Submandibular (gland) fossa

Figure 1–77
A—External oblique ridge
B—Internal oblique ridge (the anterior extension is the mylohyoid ridge)
C—Inferior cortical border of mandible
D—Submandibular (gland) fossa

Figure 1–78
A—External oblique ridge (External oblique line)
B—Internal oblique ridge (Internal oblique line)
C—Inferior cortical border of mandible
D—Submandibular fossa

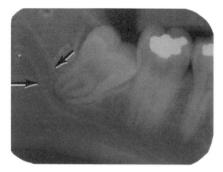

Figure 1–79
Mandibular canal (inferior alveolar canal) near apices of third molar

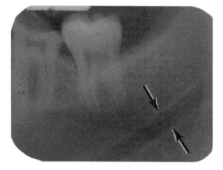

Figure 1–80
Mandibular canal (inferior alveolar canal)

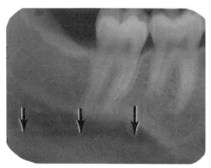

Figure 1–81
Surface of tongue

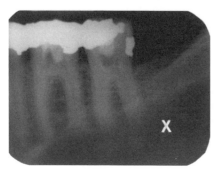

Figure 1–82
X—Submandibular fossa

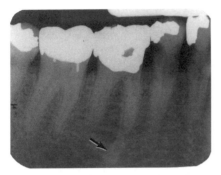

Figure 1–83

Calcification around nutrient canal leading to the apical foramen of the mesial root of the first molar

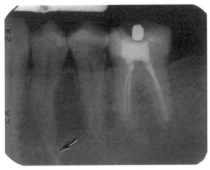

Figure 1–84

Nutrient canal leading to the apical foramen of the root of the first premolar. Presence of calcification around nutrient canal

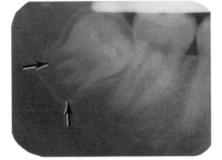

Figure 1–85

Dental papillae (Developing roots)

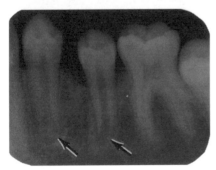

Figure 1–86

Dental papillae. The incomplete root apices persist for 1 to 2 years after the teeth have erupted

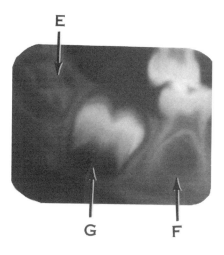

Figure 1–87

E—Calcification of cusps in the tooth follicle of the second permanent molar

F—Tooth follicle of the second premolar between the roots of the deciduous second molar

G—Dental papilla

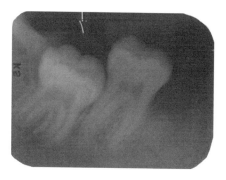

Figure 1–88

Follicular space around the crown of the unerupted third molar

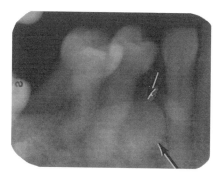

Figure 1–89

Large mandibular torus

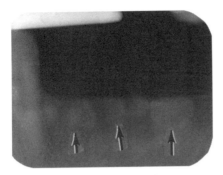

Figure 1–90
Mandibular tori (exostoses)

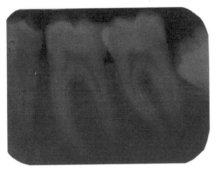

Figure 1–91
Sparse trabeculae (wide intertrabecular spaces)

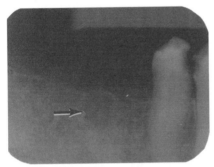

Figure 1–92
Large marrow space (wide intertrabecular space)

Also known as focal osteoporotic bone marrow defect because normal bone fails to be deposited at the extraction site. Instead, normal red or yellow bone marrow fills the area

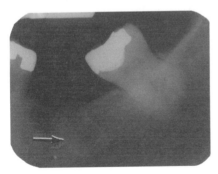

Figure 1–93
Large marrow space (wide intertrabecular space, focal osteoporotic bone marrow defect)

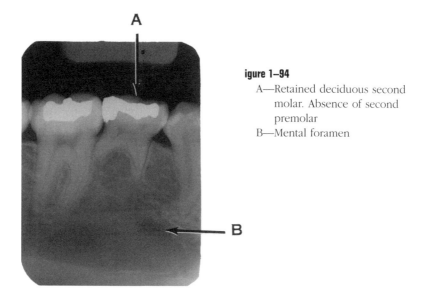

igure 1–94
A—Retained deciduous second molar. Absence of second premolar
B—Mental foramen

RESTORATIVE MATERIALS

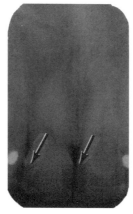

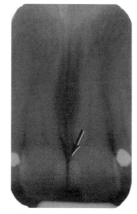

Figure 1–95
Composite resin restorations which are radiolucent may resemble caries. The well–demarcated borders differentiate them from caries

Figure 1–96
Composite resin restorations which are intentionally made opaque by manufacturers to differentiate them from caries

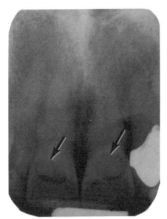

Figure 1–97

Composite resin restorations (radiolucent) which are placed on the facial or lingual surfaces of the incisor teeth. May be misdiagnosed as caries.

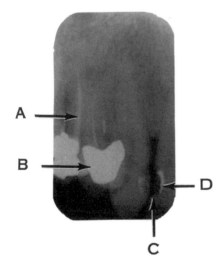

Figure 1–98

A—Gutta–percha

B—Metal coping (porcelain fused to metal)

C—Composite resin restorations (radiolucent)

D—Radiopaque liner (radiopaque calcium hydroxide) placed under composite restorations

(Commercial forms of calcium hydroxide are radiopaque whereas pure calcium hydroxide is radiolucent)

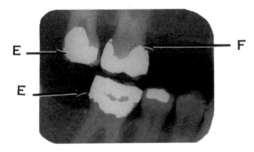

Figure 1–99

E—Silver amalgam restorations

F—Calcium hydroxide lining (radiolucent) underneath amalgam and zinc phosphate base. The commercial forms of calcium hydroxide (example, Dycal®, Life®, etc.) are radiopaque

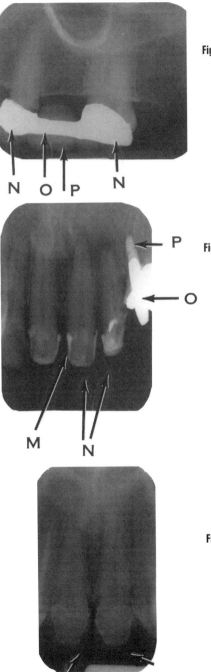

Figure 1–100
N—Metal abutments of bridge (bridge copings)
O—Gold pontic
P—Porcelain facing of pontic

Figure 1–101
M—Zinc phosphate cement
N—Acrylic jacket crown (extremely radiolucent)
O—Gold post and core
P—Gutta.percha in root canal

Figure 1–102
Porcelain jacket crown is radiolucent. Unlike acrylic which is extremely radiolucent, porcelain casts a faint image

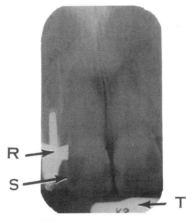

Figure 1–103

R—Gold post and core
S—Composite resin restoration
T—Metal rod of x–ray instrument

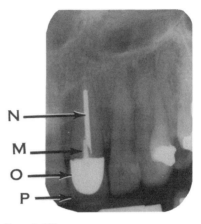

Figure 1–104

M—Metal post
N—Silver point to fill root canal
O—Metal coping
P—Porcelain crown fused to gold
core

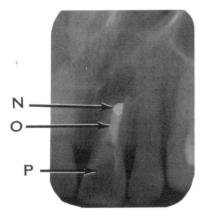

Figure 1–105

N—Retrograde amalgam filling
(silver amalgam at apex of
tooth after apicoectomy was
performed)
O—Gutta.percha in root canal
P—Composite resin restoration on
lingual surface

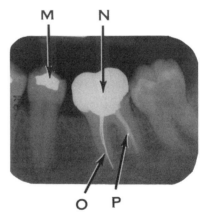

Figure 1–106

M—Silver amalgam restoration
N—Gold crown
O—Silver points
P—Gutta.Percha

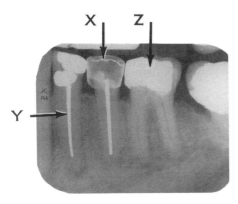

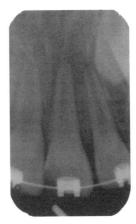

Figure 1–107

X—Prefabricated aluminum crown
Y—Silver point
Z—Amalgam with cement base

Figure 1–108
Orthodontic brackets and wire

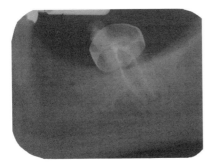

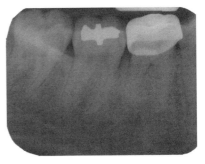

Figure 1–109
Stainless steel band on crown of molar tooth

Figure 1–110
Stainless steel crown on first molar

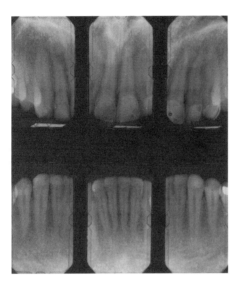

Figure 1–111

All anterior teeth are bonded with resin. The bonding was done because the teeth were affected with amelogenesis imperfecta

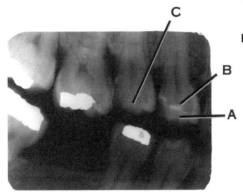

Figure 1–112

Posterior composite resin and glass ionomer cement are radiopaque. Glass ionomer cement is used as a liner and a fluoride.releasing agent to prevent recurrent caries

A—Posterior composite resin
B—Glass ionomer liner
C—Posterior composite resin

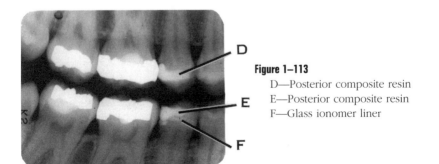

Figure 1–113

D—Posterior composite resin
E—Posterior composite resin
F—Glass ionomer liner

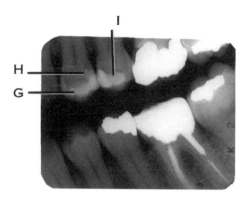

Figure 1–114

G—Posterior composite resin
H—Glass ionomer liner
I—Posterior composite resin

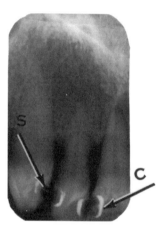

Figure 1–115

C—Zinc phosphate cement base (radiopaque) under a radiolucent restoration
S—Radiolucent restoration over a zinc phosphate cement base

Zinc phosphate and zinc oxide eugenol cements are both radiopaque. Pure calcium hydroxide cement is radiolucent but commercial forms of calcium hydroxide cement are radiopaque.

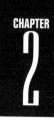

PANORAMIC ANATOMY

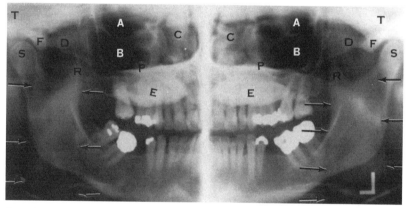

Figure 2–1

A—Orbit (Inferior portion of orbit superimposed on superior portion of maxillary sinus)

B—Maxillary sinus (antrum)

C—Nasal fossa (cavity)

D—Zygomatic arch

E—Torus palatinus (although seen twice, there is only one torus in the midline of palate)

F—Articular eminence

P—Hard palate (continues laterally on the radiograph as soft palate)

R—Coronoid process (often the pterygoid plates are superimposed on this coronoid process)

S—Condyle

T—Middle cranial fossa

Unnumbered arrows (Faint images)—Plastic or wooden vertical head stabilizers (ipsilateral side).

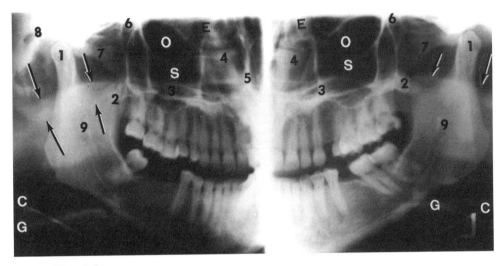

Figure 2–2

1—Condyle

2—Pterygoid plates superimposed on coronoid process

3—Hard palate. The inferior horizontal radiopaque line is the ipsilateral palate; the superior horizontal radiopaque line is the ghost image of the contralateral palate

4—Nasal concha (turbinate bone)

5—Nasal septum

6—Pterygomaxillary fissure

7—Zygomatic arch (formed by the temporal process of the zygomatic bone and zygomatic process of the temporal bone)

8—External auditory meatus

9—Mandibular foramen

Unnumbered arrows—soft palate

E—Ethmoid sinus

O—Orbit (inferior portion of orbit superimposed on superior portion of maxillary sinus)

S—Maxillary sinus

C—Horizontal chin rest (ipsilateral side)

G—Ghost image of horizontal chin rest (contralateral side)

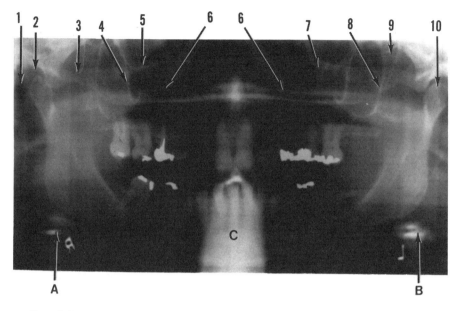

Figure 2–3

    A—Ghost (reverse) image of lead marker "L"

    B—Ghost (reverse) image of lead marker "R"

    C—Ghost image of cervical spine

    1—External auditory meatus

    2—Glenoid fossa

    3—Zygomatic arch

    4—Zygomatic process of maxilla (U-shaped)

    5—Inferior border of orbit

    6—Hard palate. The superior lines (arrows) are ghost images of contralateral
       palate; the inferior lines are the actual images of ipsilateral palate

    7—Infraorbital canal

    8—Posterolateral border of maxilla

    9—Pterygomaxillary fissure

  10—Condyle

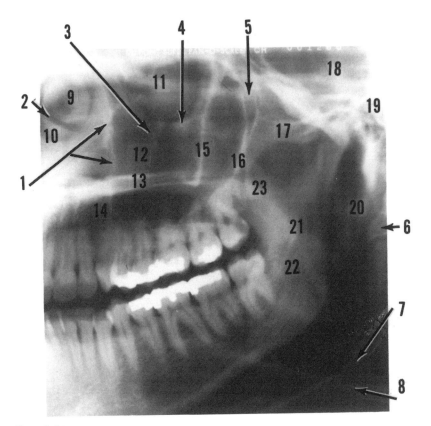

Figure 2–4

Panoramic radiograph (cut in half)
1—Lateral wall of nasal fossa
  (medial wall of maxillary sinus)
2—Middle nasal meatus
3—Infraorbital canal
4—Inferior border of orbit
5—Pterygomaxillary fissure
6—Vertebrae
7—Horizontal chin rest (ipsilateral side)
8—Ghost image of horizontal chin rest (contralateral side)
9—Middle nasal concha
10—Inferior nasal concha
11—Orbit
12—Maxillary sinus
13—Hard palate
14—Palatoglossal air space
  (between the palate and tongue)
15—Zygomatic process of maxilla
16—Posterolateral border of maxilla
17—Zygomatic arch
18—Middle cranial fossa
19—Mastoid air cells and mastoid process
20—Styloid process and ear lobe
21—Mandibular foramen
22—Mandibular canal
23—Coronoid process

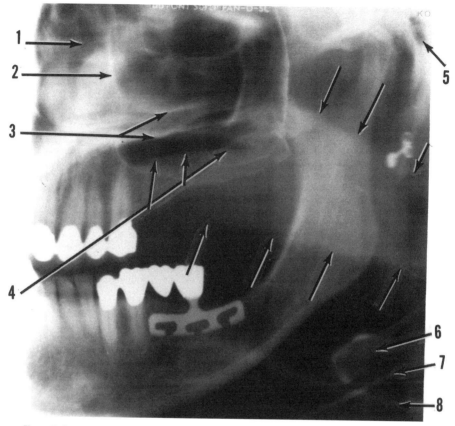

Figure 2–5

Panoramic radiograph (cut in half)

1—Nasal meatus

2—Lateral wall of nasal fossa (medial wall of maxillary sinus)

3—Hard palate. The superior arrow points at the ghost image of contralateral palate; the inferior arrow points at the image of ipsilateral palate

4—Superior surface of tongue. The radiolucency between the tongue and the hard palate is the palatoglossal air space

5—External auditory meatus

6—Hyoid bone

7—Horizontal chin rest (ipsilateral side)

8—Ghost image of horizontal chin rest (contralateral side)

Image between unnumbered arrows—ghost image of contralateral ramus

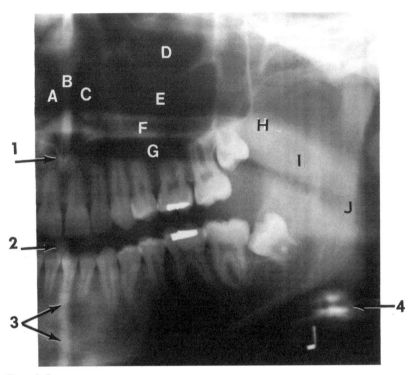

Figure 2–6

Panoramic radiograph (cut in half)

1—Anterior nasal spine
2—Bite guide (bite block)
3—Bite guide support holder
4—Ghost (reverse) image of lead marker "R" of contralateral side
A—Right nasal fossa (cavity)
B—Nasal septum
C—Left nasal fossa
D—Orbit
E—Maxillary sinus
F—Hard palate. The superior radiopaque line is the ghost image of contralateral palate whereas the inferior radiopaque line is the image of the ipsilateral palate.
G—Palatoglossal air space
H—Coronoid process. Sometimes the pterygoid plates are superimposed on the coronoid process
I—Soft palate
J—Glossopharyngeal air space

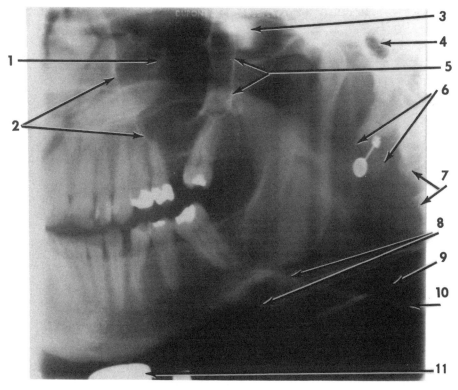

Figure 2–7

Panoramic radiograph (cut in half)

1—Infraorbital canal
2—Medial wall of maxillary sinus (lateral wall of nasal fossa)
3—Ghost image of contralateral earring
4—External auditory meatus
5—Posterolateral border of maxilla
6—Ear lobe pierced with an earring
7—Vertebrae
8—Hyoid bone
9—Horizontal chin rest (ipsilateral side)
10—Ghost image of horizontal chin rest (contralateral side)
11—Chin rest metal support holder

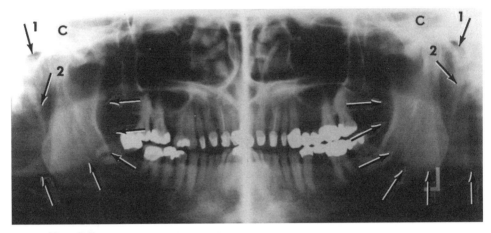

Figure 2–8

Unnumbered arrows are pointing at the ghost image of contralateral mandible

1—External auditory meatus
2—Styloid process
C—Middle cranial fossa

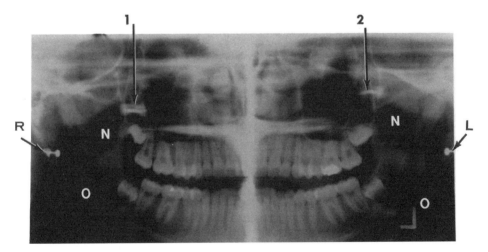

Figure 2–9

N—Nasopharynx
O—Glossopharynx
R—Earring on right ear lobe
L—Earring on left ear lobe
1—Ghost image of left earring
2—Ghost image of right earring

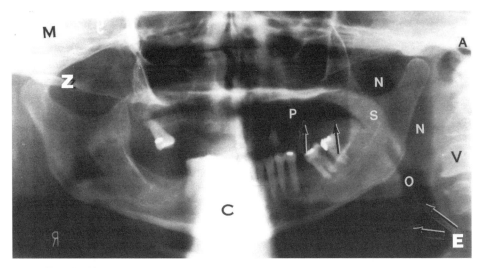

Figure 2–10A

N—Nasopharynx (superior to soft palate)

S—Soft palate

O—Glossopharynx (inferior to soft palate)

E—Epiglottis

P—Palatoglossal air space. The unnumbered two arrows under

"P" point at the surface of the tongue

C—Ghost image of cervical spine

M—Middle cranial fossa

Z—Zygomatic arch

A—External auditory meatus

V—Vertebrae

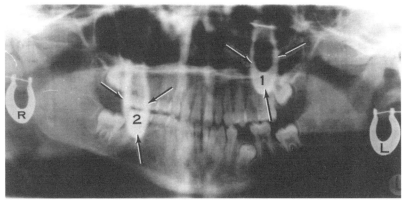

Figure 2–10B

R—Earring on right ear lobe

L—Earring on left ear lobe

1—Ghost image of right earring

2—Ghost image of left earring

Note: A ghost image is a blurry reverse image of an object that is imaged superiorly on the contralateral side.

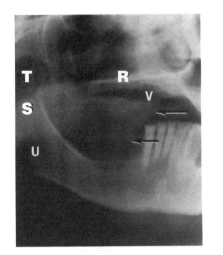
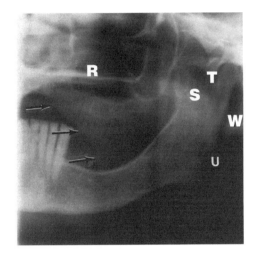

Figure 2–11
R—Hard palate (and continues laterally to form the soft palate)
S—Soft palate (which is a continuation of the hard palate)
T—Nasopharyngeal air space (superior to soft palate)
U—Glossopharyngeal air space (inferior to soft palate)
V—Palatoglossal air space (between the surface of tongue and hard palate)
W—Ear lobe
Unnumbered arrows—Nasolabial folds (cheeks)

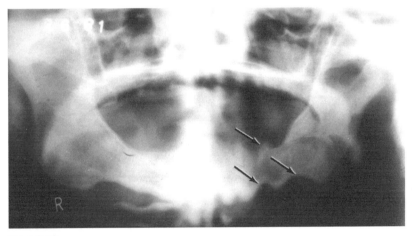

Figure 2–12
The panoramic radiograph shows indentations of the body of the mandible (arrows). It was imaged while the patient had hiccups, resulting in upward movements of the jaws. A similar image is produced when the patient chews gum during x-ray exposure.

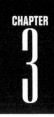

PATIENT POSITIONING ERRORS IN PANORAMIC RADIOGRAPHY

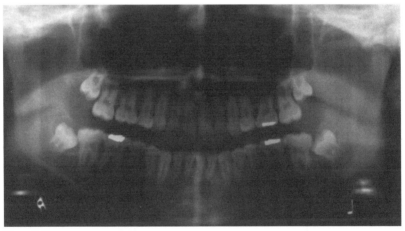

Figure 3–1

Correct positioning of patient's head in the panoramic machine. Note the slight downward curvative of the occlusal plane and the untilted vertical rami. Notice the sharpness of images of the anterior teeth.

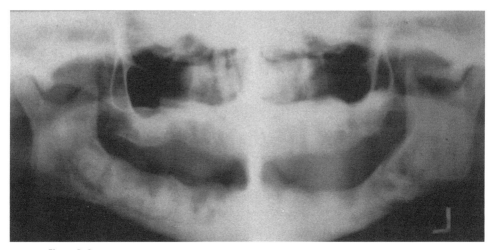

Figure 3–2
Edentulous patient. Correct positioning of patient's head in the panoramic machine. Note the slight downward curvature of the occlusal plane and the untilted vertical rami. The lesion in the jaws is florid osseous dysplasia (diffuse cementosis).

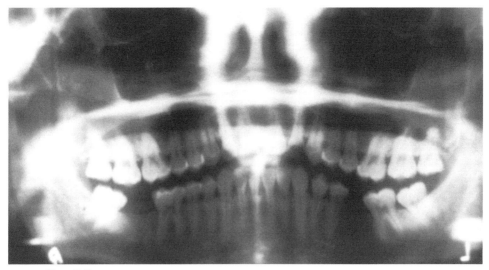

Figure 3–3
Patient's head is tilted backwards; that is, the chin is positioned upwards. Note the downward curvature of the occlusal plane. The rami are tilted laterally. The palate is superimposed on the apices of the maxillary incisors.

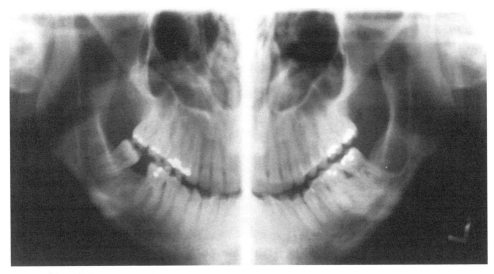

Figure 3–4
Patient's head is tilted downwards; that is, the chin is positioned too low.
Note the upward curvature of the occlusal plane. The rami are tilted medially.

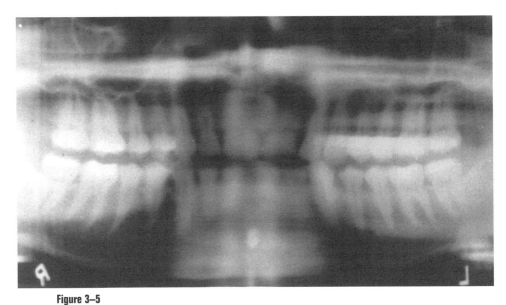

Figure 3–5
Patient's teeth are positioned posterior to the focal trough (zone of sharpness).
Note the horizontal magnification and unsharpness of anterior teeth.

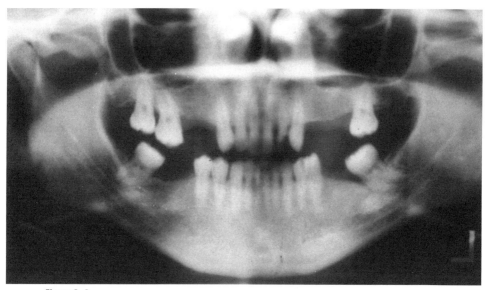

Figure 3–6

Patient's teeth are positioned anterior to the focal trough (zone of sharpness). Note the horizontal demagnification and unsharpness of anterior teeth.

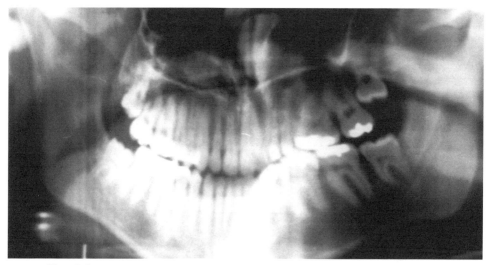

Figure 3–7

Patient's head is positioned towards one side (laterally) and outside of the focal trough (zone of sharpness); that is, the patient's mid-sagittal plane is not positioned in the middle of the two head positioners. One side of the jaws is horizontally demagnified while the other side is magnified.

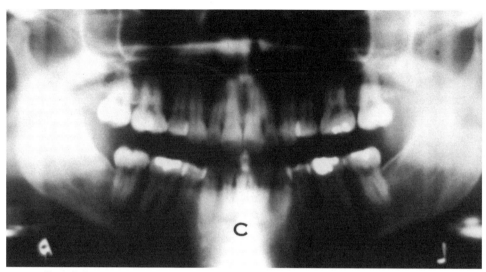

Figure 3–8

Patient's neck is not in an erect position, that is, the patient is stooping. The ghost image of the cervical spine (C) produces a broad radiopacity in the midline.

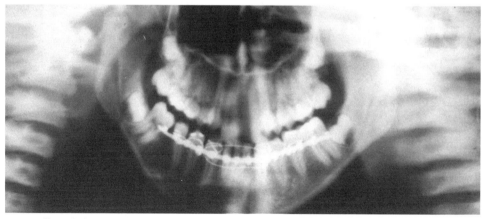

Figure 3–9

Patient's head and neck are placed excessively forward in the panoramic machine resulting in bilateral prominent images of the vertebrae. The vertebrae are prominently seen whenever the neck is positioned too forward. The anterior teeth are horizontally demagnified and unsharp. The patient's head is also tilted downwards. Note the upward curvature of the occlusal plane and the medial tilt of the rami.

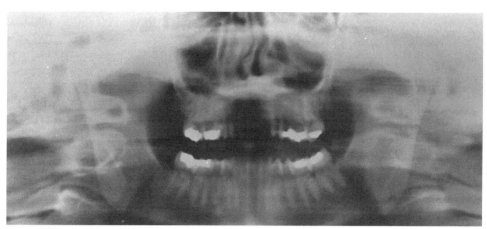

Figure 3–10A

Patient's teeth are positioned anterior to the focal trough. The excessive anterior positioning has produced horizontal demagnification, giving the illusion of missing anterior teeth.

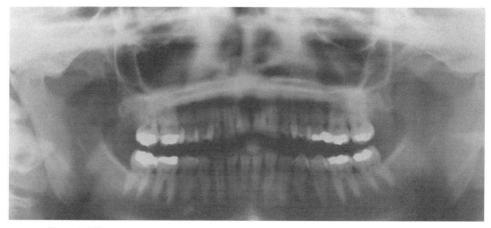

Figure 3–10B

The same patient when teeth are positioned in the focal trough results in the visibility of all the anterior teeth. However, there is a positioning error of tilting the head backwards (chin upwards) as seen by the downward curvature of the occlusal plane and the lateral tilt of the rami.

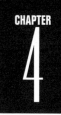

EXTRAORAL AND OCCLUSAL ANATOMIC LANDMARKS

LATERAL SKULL RADIOGRAPH

(FIGURES 4–1 TO 4–4)

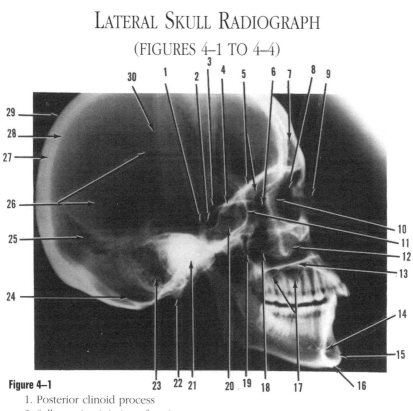

Figure 4–1

1. Posterior clinoid process
2. Sella turcica (pituitary fossa)
3. Anterior clinoid process
4. Floor of anterior cranial fossa in the midline

5. Orbital plates of frontal bone (Roof of orbit and floor of anterior cranial fossa lateral to midline)
6. Ethmoid sinus
7. Frontal sinus
8. Orbit
9. Nasal bones
10. Lateral border of orbit (formed by frontal process of zygoma and zygomatic process of frontal bone)
11. Greater wing of sphenoid bone forming anterior wall of middle cranial fossa
12. Zygomatic process of maxilla (U-shaped)
13. Hard palate forming floor of nasal fossa
14. Lingual cortical plate of anterior portion of mandible
15. Buccal cortical plate of anterior portion of mandible
16. Mentum
17. Floor of maxillary sinus
18. Zygoma (arrow points at inferior border of zygoma)
19. Pterygomaxillary fissure
20. Sphenoid sinus
21. Petrous portion of temporal bone
22. Mastoid process of temporal bone
23. Mastoid air cells
24. Floor of posterior cranial fossa
25. Lambdoid suture
26. Markings of middle meningeal vessels
27. Diploe
28. Inner table of bone
29. Outer table of bone
30. Posterior border of ear plug holder of cephalostat

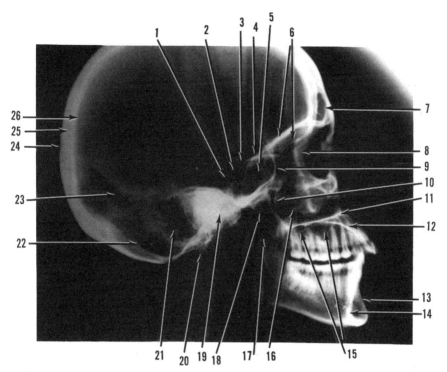

Figure 4–2

1. Posterior clinoid process
2. Sella turcica (pituitary fossa)
3. Anterior clinoid process
4. Floor of anterior cranial fossa in the midline
5. Sphenoid sinus
6. Orbital plates of frontal bone (Roof of orbit and floor of anterior cranial fossa lateral to midline)
7. Frontal sinus
8. Lateral border of orbit (formed by frontal process of zygoma and zygomatic process of frontal bone)
9. Greater wing of the sphenoid bone forming the anterior wall of the middle cranial fossa
10. Pterygomaxillary fissure
11. Hard palate forming floor of nasal fossa
12. Roof of palate (midline)
13. Buccal cortical plate of anterior portion of mandible
14. Lingual cortical plate of anterior portion of mandible
15. Floor of maxillary sinus
16. Zygoma (arrow points at lower border of zygoma)
17. Sigmoid notch (mandibular notch)
18. Lateral pterygoid plate
19. Petrous portion of temporal bone
20. Mastoid process of temporal bone
21. Mastoid air cells
23. Lambdoid suture
24. Outer table of bone
25. Diploe
26. Inner table of bone

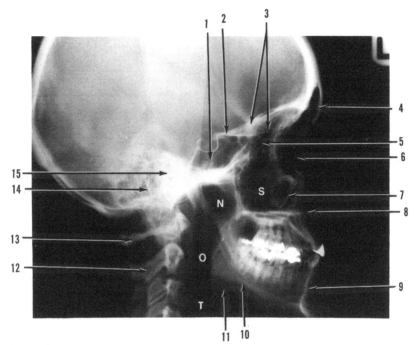

Figure 4–3

S—Maxillary sinus

N—Nasopharynx

O—Oropharynx (the anterior border is the pharyngeal surface of the base of tongue)

T—Tracheaoesophageal space (actually starts much lower than indicated here)

1—Sphenoid sinus

2—Floor of anterior cranial fossa in the midline

3—Orbital plates of frontal bone (Roof of orbit and floor of anterior cranial fossa lateral to midline)

4—Frontal sinus

5—Ethmoid sinus

6—Orbit

7—Zygomatic processes of maxilla (one is of the side closer to the film and the other is of the side farther from the film)

8—Anterior nasal spine

9—Lingual cortical plate of anterior portion of mandible

10—Lower border of mandible of side closer to the film

11—Lower border of mandible of side farther from the film

12—Axis (second cervical vertebra)

13—Atlas (first cervical vertebra)

14—Mastoid air cells

15—Petrous portion of the temporal bone

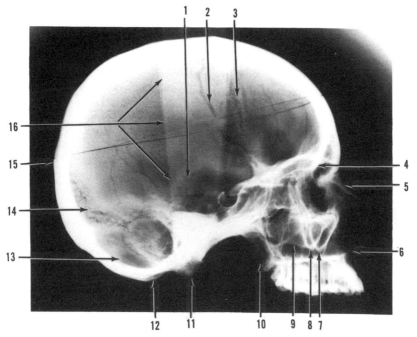

Figure 4–4

1. Squamoparietal suture
2. Markings of the middle meningeal vessels
3. Coronal suture
4. Supraorbital margin
5. Nasal bones
6. Anterior nasal spine
7. Zygomatic process of maxilla (U-shaped) of side farther from the film
8. Zygomatic process of maxilla (U-shaped) of side closer to the film
9. Lower border of zygoma
10. Lateral pterygoid plate
11. Mastoid process of temporal bone
12. Posterior border of foramen magnum
13. Floor of posterior cranial fossa
14. Lambdoid suture
15. Lambda
16. Posterior border of ear plug holder of cephalostat

POSTERO-ANTERIOR RADIOGRAPH
(FIGURE 4–5 TO 4–8)

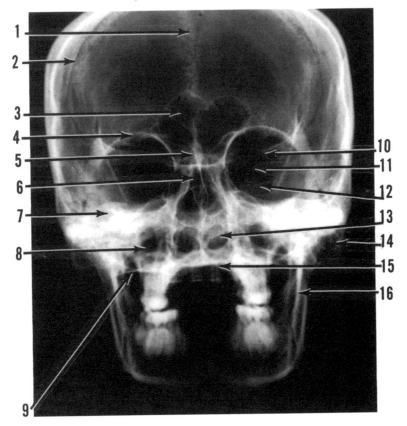

Figure 4–5

1. Sagittal suture
2. Coronal suture
3. Frontal sinus
4. Superior border of orbit
5. Crista galli
6. Sphenoid sinus
7. Petrous portion of temporal bone
8. Maxillary sinus
9. Floor of posterior cranial fossa

10. Lesser wing of sphenoid
11. Superior orbital fissure
12. Greater wing of sphenoid
13. Nasal cavity
14. Mastoid process and mastoid air cells
15. Floor of nasal fossa (hard palate)
16. External oblique ridge

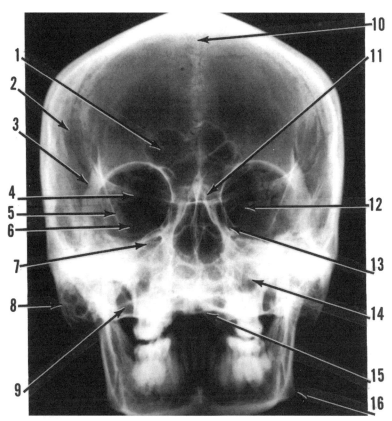

Figure 4–6

1. Frontal sinus
2. Coronal suture
3. Zygomatic process of frontal bone (joins to frontal process of zygomatic bone)
4. Lesser wing of sphenoid
5. Squamozygomatic surface of greater wing of sphenoid (innominate line)
6. Greater wing of sphenoid
7. Infraorbital foramen
8. Mastoid process and mastoid air cells
9. Zygomatic process of maxilla
10. Bregma
11. Ethmoid sinus (ethmoid air cells)
12. Superior orbital fissure
13. Lacrimal canal (nasolacrimal canal)
14. Maxillary sinus
15. Floor of nasal fossa (hard palate)
16. Gonion

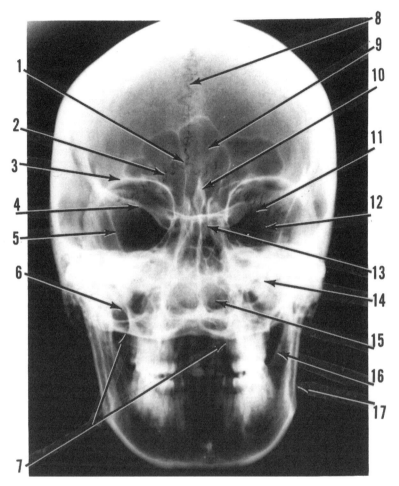

Figure 4–7 Antero-Posterior Radiograph

1. Lambda
2. Lambdoid suture
3. Superior border of orbit
4. Lesser wing of sphenoid
5. Squamozygomatic surface of greater wing of sphenoid (innominate line)
6. Zygomatic process of maxilla
7. Floor of posterior cranial fossa
8. Sagittal suture
9. Frontal sinus
10. Crista galli
11. Superior orbital fissure
12. Greater wing of sphenoid
13. Sphenoid sinus
14. Petrous portion of temporal bone
15. Nasal cavity
16. Anterior border of ramus
17. Posterior border of ramus

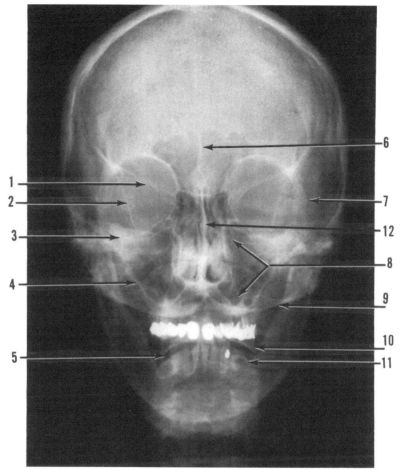

Figure 4–8

1. Lesser wing of sphenoid
2. Squamozygomatic surface of greater wing of sphenoid
3. Petrous portion of temporal bone
4. Zygomatic process of maxilla
5. Atlas—axis articulation
6. Frontal crest
7. Zygomatic process of frontal bone (joins to frontal process of zygomatic bone)
8. Maxillary sinus
9. Floor of posterior cranial fossa
10. Transverse process of atlas
11. Transverse process of axis
12. Nasal septum (composed of the perpendicular plate of the ethmoid bone and the vomer bone)

SUBMENTO-VERTEX RADIOGRAPH
(FIGURE 4–9 TO 4–10)

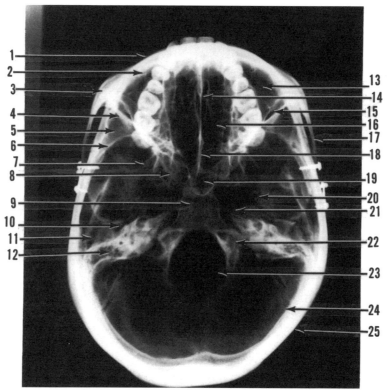

Figure 4–9

(Mandible has been removed for better visualization of the base of the skull)

1. Outer cortical plate of frontal bone
2. Inner cortical plate of frontal bone
3. Body of zygoma
4. Lateral wall of orbit (greater wing of sphenoid)
5. Infratemporal surface of greater wing of sphenoid
6. Anterior wall of middle cranial fossa formed by the greater wing of sphenoid
7. Lateral pterygoid plate
8. Medial pterygoid plate
9. Clivus
10. Eustachian canal (internal auditory canal)
11. External auditory canal
12. Petrous portion of temporal bone
13. Maxillary sinus (superimposed on orbit)
14. Nasal septum (perpendicular plate of ethmoid)
15. Inferior orbital fissure
16. Ethmoid air cells opening into nasal fossa

17. Zygomatic arch
18. Posterior border of vomer (part of nasal septum)
19. Sphenoid sinus
20. Foramen spinosum
21. Foramen lacerum

22. Occipital condyle
23. Foramen magnum
24. Inner cortical plate of occipital bone
25. Outer cortical plate of occipital bone

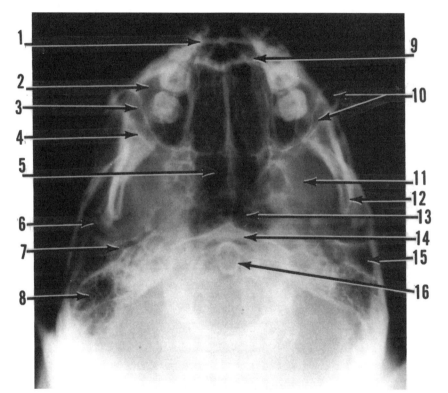

Figure 4–10

1. Superior (alveolar) border of mandible
2. Maxillary sinus
3. Lateral wall of maxillary sinus
4. Lateral wall of orbit (greater wing of sphenoid)
5. Sphenoid sinus
6. Mandibular condyle
7. Eustachian canal (internal auditory canal)
8. Mastoid air cells
9. Inferior border of mandible
10. Inferior orbital fissure
11. Middle cranial fossa
12. Coronoid process
13. Clivus
14. Anterior arch of first cervical vertebra
15. External auditory canal
16. Odontoid process (dens) of axis

WATERS' VIEW
(POSTERO-ANTERIOR MAXILLARY SINUS RADIOGRAPH)
(FIGURE 4–11 TO 4–12)

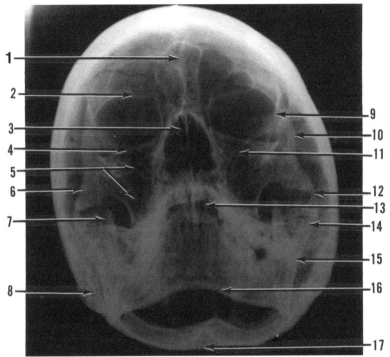

Figure 4–11

1. Frontal sinus
2. Supraorbital notch
3. Ethmoid sinus
4. Anterior margin of orbital floor
5. Maxillary sinus
6. Body of zygoma
7. Coronoid process
8. Mastoid air cells
9. Squamozygomatic surface of greater wing of sphenoid (innominate line)
10. Frontal process of zygoma (joins the zygomatic process of frontal bone)
11. Lesser wing of sphenoid (the radiolucent line is the superior orbital fissure)
12. Zygomatic arch
13. Sphenoid sinus
14. Condyle
15. Ramus of mandible
16. Inferior border of body of mandible
17. Inferior aspect of base of skull

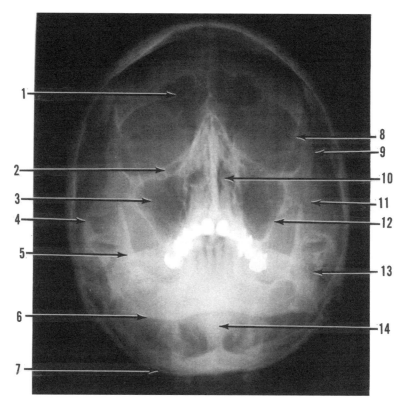

Figure 4–12
1. Frontal sinus
2. Infraorbital foramen and canal
3. Maxillary sinus
4. Zygomatic arch
5. Floor of middle cranial fossa
6. Inferior border of body of mandible
7. Inferior aspect of base of skull
8. Squamozygomatic surface of greater wing of sphenoid
9. Frontal process of zygoma
10. Nasal fossa and conchae (turbinates)
11. Body of zygoma
12. Lateral wall of maxillary sinus
13. Ramus of mandible
14. Odontoid process of axis

TRANSCRANIAL RADIOGRAPH OF TEMPOROMANDIBULAR JOINT
(FIGURE 4–13 TO 4–16)

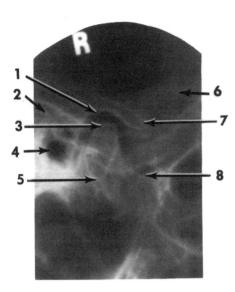

Figure 4–13

Closed mouth position (transcranial projection)

1. Glenoid fossa (articular fossa)
2. Mastoid air cells
3. Lateral pole of condyle
4. External auditory meatus
5. Medial pole of condyle
6. Zygomatic process of temporal bone
7. Articular tubercle (articular eminence)
8. Sigmoid notch (mandibular notch)

The space between the lateral pole of the condyle and the glenoid fossa is the joint space which contains the articular disc. The articular disc is not visible on a radiograph because it is radiolucent.

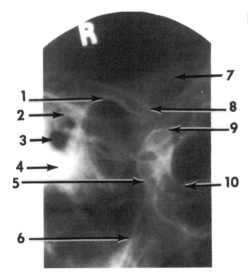

Figure 4–14

Open mouth position (transcranial projection)

1. Glenoid fossa (articular fossa)
2. Mastoid air cells
3. External auditory meatus
4. Mastoid process
5. Medial pole of condyle
6. Posterior border of ramus of mandible
7. Zygomatic process of temporal bone
8. Articular tubercle (articular eminence)
9. Lateral pole of condyle
10. Sigmoid notch (mandibular notch)

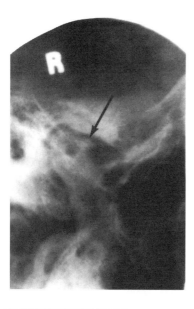

Figure 4–15

Osteoarthritis

Transcranial radiograph showing: (a) osteophyte (lipping) indicated by arrow; (b) flattened condyle; (c) reduced joint space; (d) flattened posterior slope of the articular eminence; (e) shallowed articular fossa.

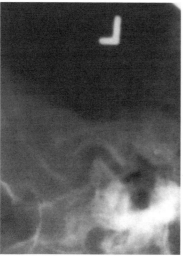

Figure 4–16

Advanced stage of rheumatoid arthritis. Transcranial radiograph showing a "sharpened pencil" deformity due to extensive erosion of the condyle.

OCCLUSAL RADIOGRAPH
(FIGURE 4–17 TO 4–22)

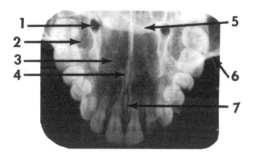

Figure 4–17

Maxillary occlusal radiograph

1. Nasolacrimal canal (orbital entrance) superimposed on posterior surface of hard palate
2. Maxillary sinus
3. Nasal fossa
4. Nasal septum
5. Superciliary arch (forehead)
6. Zygomatic process of maxilla
7. Incisive foramen

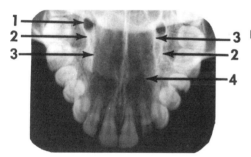

Figure 4–18

Maxillary occlusal radiograph

1. Nasolacrimal canal
2. Medial wall of maxillary sinus
3. Lateral wall of nasal fossa
4. Nasal fossa

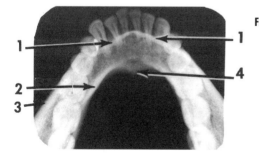

Figure 4–19

Mandibular occlusal radiograph

1. Mental ridges
2. Internal oblique ridge (mylohyoid ridge)
3. Inferior border of mandible (cortical bone)
4. Genial tubercles

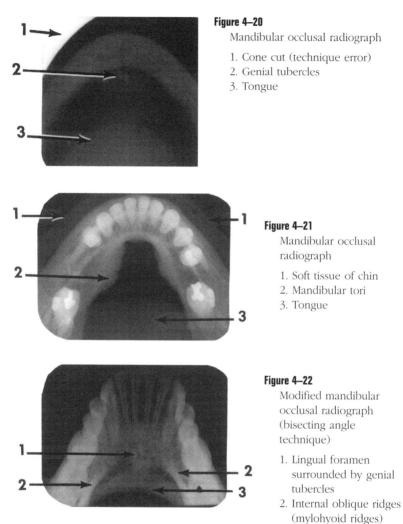

Figure 4–20

Mandibular occlusal radiograph

1. Cone cut (technique error)
2. Genial tubercles
3. Tongue

Figure 4–21

Mandibular occlusal radiograph

1. Soft tissue of chin
2. Mandibular tori
3. Tongue

Figure 4–22

Modified mandibular occlusal radiograph (bisecting angle technique)

1. Lingual foramen surrounded by genial tubercles
2. Internal oblique ridges (mylohyoid ridges)
3. Inferior border of mandible (cortical bone)

DENTAL CARIES

Radiographic interpretation of dental caries should always be undertaken with a clinical examination of the oral cavity. Caries is detected radiographically only in the advanced stages when there is sufficient decalcification of tooth structures. The radiographic appearance of caries is not representative of its actual size; that is, it is much larger clinically than seen on a radiograph. Initial carious lesions are not readily visualized on a radiograph because the visibility of caries is determined by the ratio of enamel to caries through which xrays penetrate. Although bite-wing radiographs are more useful in caries detection, the importance of periapical radiographs should not be underestimated. The treatment of a carious tooth should not be based on a single radiograph because an incorrect horizontal or vertical angulation of the x-ray beam can result in a number of illusions. Also, errors in exposure factors and errors in processing can produce radiographic illusions of dental caries. A radiographic diagnosis of caries must always be supplemented with a careful clinical examination.

OCCLUSAL CARIES

Occlusal caries originates in the pits and fissures of premolar and molar teeth. When caries is still in the enamel, there is no radiographic evidence of occlusal caries. At this stage, it can only be detected by a careful clinical examination with an explorer. Occlusal caries is observed radiographically only after the decay process has penetrated the enamel fissures to the dentino-enamel junction. Here, the caries spreads and, on a radiograph, shows a radiolucent line at the dentino-enamel junction. This spread of caries along the junction may undermine the enamel cusps and fracture them from the tooth. Histopathologically, the spread of caries in the enamel follows the path of the enamel rods and produces a triangular appearance with the base of the triangle at the dentino-enamel junction and the apex of the triangle towards the occlusal surface of the tooth. In the dentin, the occlusal caries follows the path of the dentinal tubules and forms another triangular radiolucency but with the base of the triangle at the dentino-enamel junction and the apex towards the dental pulp. Thus, occlusal caries progresses to form two triangular areas with a common base at the dentino-enamel junction. It must be noted that the tendency for dentinal caries to be restricted by the path of the tubules is not absolute, such that large carious lesions in the dentin give a diffuse appearance as they expand towards the pulp. The diffuse periphery of occlusal caries differentiates it from facial and lingual caries.

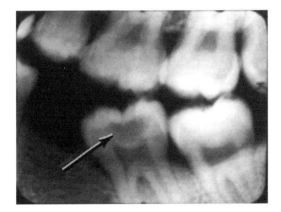

Figure 5–1

    Occlusal caries on a mandibular molar. Notice the intact enamel surface. Also observe the diffuse triangular appearance of the caries with the base of the triangle at the dentino-enamel junction and the apex towards the dental pulp.

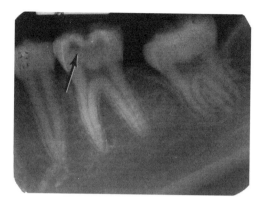

Figure 5-2

Occlusal caries in the first molar. Occlusal caries spreads at the dentino-enamel junction and may undermine and fracture the enamel. In the enamel, caries progresses in the direction of the enamel rods; in the dentin, caries progresses in the direction of the dentinal tubules.

PROXIMAL CARIES

Proximal caries is initially detected on a radiograph by a small notching on the enamel surface just below the proximal contact point. Histopathologically, as the carious lesion in the enamel follows the path of the enamel rods and increases in size, it continues to demonstrate approximately a triangular pattern with its base towards the outer surface of the tooth and with a flattened apex towards the dentino-enamel junction. After reaching the dentino-enamel junction, the carious lesion spreads along the junction and forms a second base. From this second base, the caries proceeds towards the pulp along the path of the dentinal tubules and forms another triangular radiolucency with the apex towards the pulp. Thus, proximal caries progresses to form two triangular areas with the base of the first triangle at the outer enamel surface of the tooth and the base of the second triangle at the dentino-enamel junction. When the undermined enamel fractures, the entire carious lesion radiographically resembles a U-shape.

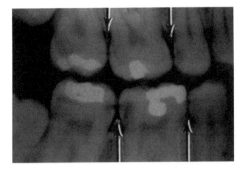

Figure 5–3

Proximal caries on maxillary and mandibular second premolars, first molars and second molars. Caries is much larger clinically than seen on the radiograph.

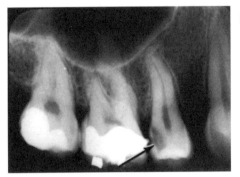

Figure 5–4

Proximal caries on the distal surface of the second premolar. Notice the triangular appearance of caries. In the enamel, caries progresses along the path of the enamel rods; in the dentin, caries progresses roughly along the path of the dentinal tubules.

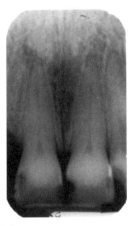
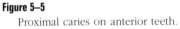

Figure 5–5

Proximal caries on anterior teeth.

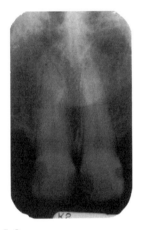

Figure 5–6

Radiolucent restorative materials (composite resin) may be misdiagnosed as caries. Notice the box-like rectangular cavity preparations.

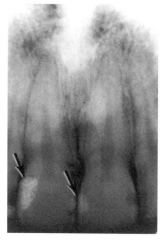

Figure 5–7

Radiopaque particles added to radiolucent restorative materials (composite resin) by manufacturer to differentiate them from carious lesions.

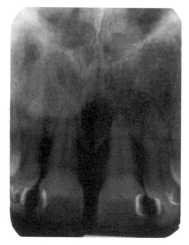

Figure 5–8

The radiopaque cement bases underneath the radiolucent restorations differentiates them from carious lesions.

FACIAL AND LINGUAL CARIES

Facial and lingual (palatal) caries originate in pits and grooves on the facial and lingual surfaces. Similar to occlusal and proximal caries, the facial and lingual caries histopathologically tend to follow the path of the enamel rods and dentinal tubules. The radiographic radiolucency is well-demarcated from the surrounding sound tooth structure. Its shape may be round, oval or semilunar, and depends on its location and degree of extension. Carious lesions developing in the facial and lingual pits are usually round (or oval) while those at the free margin of the gingiva are round (or oval) in the initial stages, but become elliptical or semilunar as they increase in size. Even after the carious lesion has penetrated the dentino-enamel junction and has spread along the junction, the undermined enamel tends to retain its integrity and provides a definite periphery to the lesion. This sharp demarcation differentiates facial and lingual caries from occlusal caries. Radiographs are useful in making a clinician aware of the presence of a lesion but its actual location and extent is determined through clinical examination. Facial caries can be differentiated radiographically from lingual caries by changing the angulations of the x-ray beam. However, this is of academic interest only and, therefore, no attempt is made to differentiate facial caries from lingual caries on a radiograph.

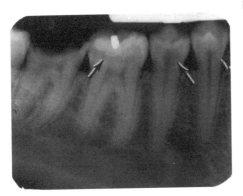

Figure 5–9

Facial or lingual caries on first and second premolars (round or oval), and on first molar (semilunar). Facial and lingual caries usually originate in pits or grooves and later spread at the dentino-enamel junction. Enamel caries tends to follow the lines of the enamel rods; dentinal caries tends to roughly follow the lines of the dentinal tubules. The whole crown of the second molar is carious.

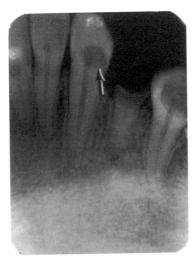

Figure 5–10

Facial or lingual caries on the canine. Facial and lingual caries are usually well-demarcated from the surrounding sound enamel. This clear-cut outline assists in differentiating such lesions from occlusal caries. The crowns of the first and second premolars are carious.

ROOT CARIES (CEMENTAL CARIES)

Root caries (cemental caries) develops between the cemento-enamel junction and the free margin of the gingiva. It does not occur in areas covered by a well-attached gingiva. Histopathologically, root caries does not follow any specific path; it simply invades the cementum and dentin of the root. On a radiograph, root caries produces a saucer-shaped (scooped-out) appearance. The carious lesion has a diffuse periphery. Frequently, root caries may be erroneously interpreted as cervical burnout, especially when the radiolucency occurs under the proximal step of a metallic restoration. For root caries to occur, there must be loss of crestal bone resulting in the exposure of cementum. Cervical burnout is discussed later in this chapter.

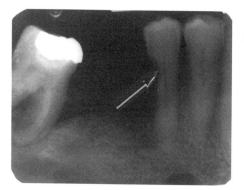

Figure 5–11

Root caries (cemental caries) on distal of second premolar. Root caries is usually saucer-shaped. Root caries does not occur in areas covered by a well-attached gingiva. There is loss of bone, resulting in the exposure of cementum.

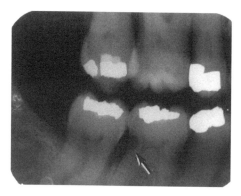

Figure 5–12

Root caries (cemental caries) on mandibular first molar has a scooped-out appearance. There is loss of alveolar bone height, resulting in the exposure of cementum.

RECURRENT CARIES

Recurrent caries is that which recurs in a previously treated and restored tooth. The caries may occur under a restoration or along its margins. If recurrent caries occurs under the proximal step of a metallic restoration, it may be misdiagnosed as cervical burnout. As the recurrent caries progresses closer to the pulp, a layer of secondary dentin may sometimes form to protect the pulp from the carious lesion. Recurrent caries may sometimes be misdiagnosed as (the noncommercial paste of) calcium hydroxide lining used underneath an amalgam and zinc phosphate base. On a radiograph, noncommercial calcium hydroxide (that is, a mixture of pure calcium hydroxide and water) produces a thin radiolucent line whereas recurrent caries produces a diffuse radiolucency. A definitive differentiation can be made only after the removal of the restoration.

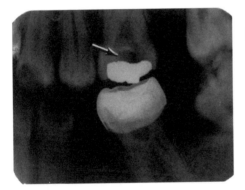

Figure 5–13
Recurrent caries underneath the amalgam restoration of the maxillary first molar. Presence of secondary dentin (radiopaque) between the recurrent caries and the pulp chamber.

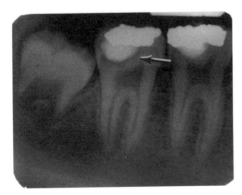

Figure 5–14
In the second molar, the diffuse radiolucent line between the zinc phosphate base and sound dentin may be either recurrent caries or calcium hydroxide lining. Clinically, after removal of the restoration, the radiolucency was diagnosed as recurrent caries.

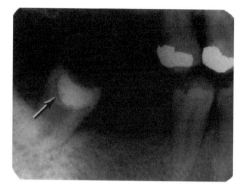

Figure 5–15
Calcium hydroxide (thin radiolucent line) between the pulp chamber and zinc phosphate cement in the molar.

CERVICAL BURNOUT

Cervical burnout is an illusion of radiolucency of a radiopaque object. It appears as a radiolucent area or band between two extremely radiopaque areas. For example, the area between the crown and that portion of the root covered by the alveolar bone absorbs fewer x-ray photons than do the adjoining areas. Cervical burnout is also produced by root configuration, shape of the cemento-enamel contour, and exposure factors (peripheral burnout). Burnout due to excessive exposure is called peripheral burnout. Cervical burnout should not be mistaken for root caries or with caries under the proximal step of a Class II restoration. Root caries occurs when the free margin of the gingiva has receded from its normal position. The occurrence of cervical burnout depends partially on the presence of alveolar bone to provide the necessary contrast. The final confirmation must be done clinically with the use of an explorer. A second radiograph made with a slightly different x-ray beam angulation and a change in exposure factors will enable the clinician to differentiate a cervical burnout from root caries.

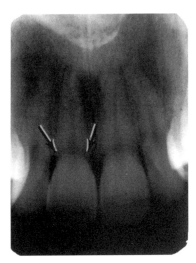

Figure 5–16A

Cervical burnout (radiolucent band) near the necks of the central incisors. Such burnout is the result of a decrease in total structural thickness and/or a change in the hard tissue composition.

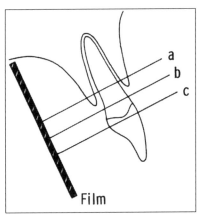

Figure 5–16B

Diagram illustrating the phenomenon of cervical burnout. Lines "a" and "c" penetrate more dense tissue than does line "b". Xray "b" penetrates tooth structures (cementum and dentin). Xray "a" penetrates tooth structures and alveolar bone. Xray "c" penetrates tooth structures and enamel. Cervical burnout can also be caused by root configuration and the shape of the cemento-enamel contour.

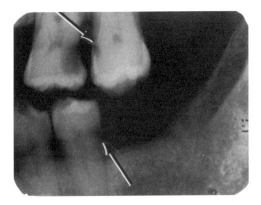

Figure 5–17

Cervical burnout and root caries. The distal surface of the mandibular second premolar and the mesial surface of the maxillary second molar (arrows) show cervical burnout whereas the distal of the maxillary first molar shows root caries.

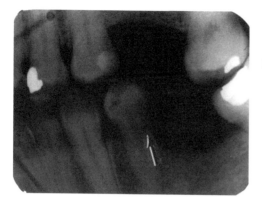

Figure 5–18A
Cervical burnout on distal of mandibular first premolar.

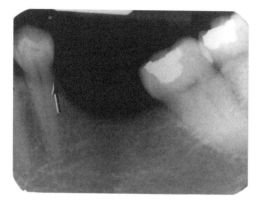

Figure 5–18B
Disappearance of cervical burnout when x-ray beam angulation and exposure are changed.

BEAM ANGULATION EFFECTS ON CARIES

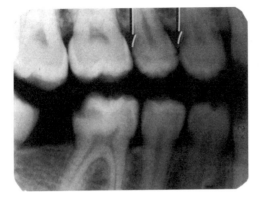

Figure 5–19
Caries visibility is usually better on a bite-wing than on a periapical radiograph.

Figure A
Bite-wing clearly shows the proximal caries on the maxillary second premolar.

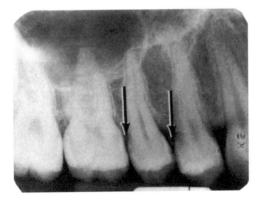

Figure B
On the periapical radiograph, the proximal caries is not as clearly visible as on the bite-wing.

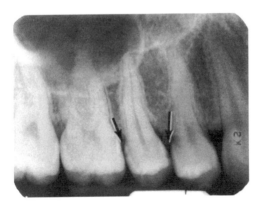

Figure 5–20
Caries visibility is better using a paralleling technique than with a bisecting angle technique.

Figure A
Paralleling technique. The proximal caries on the second premolar is clearly visible.

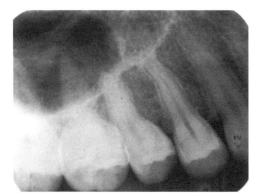

Figure B

Bisecting angle technique. The proximal caries on the second premolar is not visible.

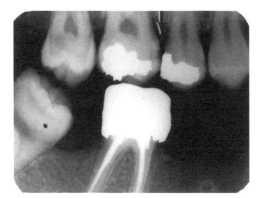

Figure 5–21A

Correct horizontal x-ray beam angulation (no overlapping) results in the detection of proximal caries on the mesial of the maxillary first molar.

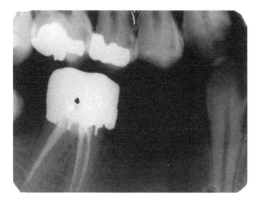

Figure 5–21B

Incorrect horizontal angulation (overlapping) results in obliteration of the proximal caries. The arrow shows the overlapping between the premolars.

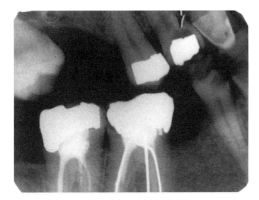

Figure 5–22

Obliteration of carious lesion when using different vertical angulations of the x-ray beam. Caries is visible on bite-wing but not on periapical radiograph.

Figure A

On the bite-wing, the recurrent caries is visible under the amalgam restoration of the maxillary first premolar.

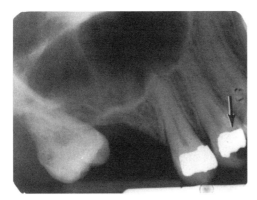

Figure B

On the periapical radiograph, the recurrent caries is not clearly visible because of an increase in the positive vertical angulation of the x-ray beam.

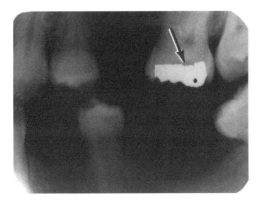

Figure 5–23

Obliteration of carious lesion when using different vertical angulations of the x-ray beam. Caries visible on periapical radiograph but not on bite-wing.

Figure A

Unlike the previous example (Fig. 5–22), this bite-wing does not show the recurrent caries under the amalgam restoration of the maxillary molar.

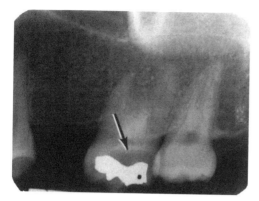

Figure B

The periapical radiograph shows the recurrent caries under the amalgam restoration. Unlike the previous example (Fig. 5–22), this periapical radiograph proved to be superior to the bite-wing in the detection of recurrent caries.

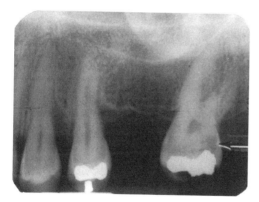

Figure 5–24

Changes in location of a carious lesion with changes in horizontal angulation of the x-ray beam.

Figure A

The recurrent caries in the molar is visible near the distal surface of the tooth.

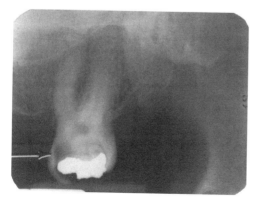

Figure B

The recurrent caries is now visible near the mesial surface of the tooth because of the change in horizontal angulation of the x-ray beam. Actually, the whole buccal surface is carious.

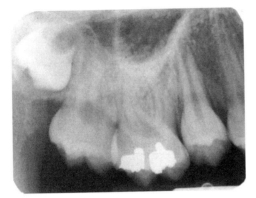

Figure 5–25
Decrease in the number of amalgam restorations with changes in horizontal angulation of the x-ray beam.

Figure A
Presence of two amalgam restorations in the first molar.

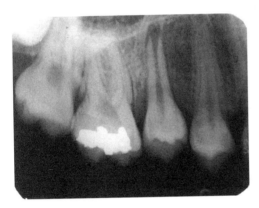

Figure B
Illusion of one amalgam restoration because of a change in the horizontal angulation of the x-ray beam.

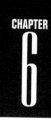

PERIODONTAL DISEASE

Although a radiograph cannot show the soft tissue changes that occur in the periodontium, it is of value when used as an adjunct to clinical findings. In spite of the association of a periodontal pocket and bone loss, the radiographic interpretation of bone loss should never be described as pocket formation. Bone loss can occur without pocket formation or may be out of proportion to the depth of the periodontal pocket when measured clinically. Visualization of the depth of a pocket may be aided by inserting a gutta-percha point into the pocket. The gutta-percha point will follow the defect because it is relatively inflexible and will appear on a radiograph because of its radiopacity. Radiographs are useful in evaluating the location of bone loss, the amount of bone loss, the direction of bone loss, the type of crestal bone irregularities, and the prognosis of the healing process. Radiographs are also useful in determining the causative irritants such as calculus, overhanging restorations, impacted foreign bodies, etc. It must be emphasized that x-ray beam angulation, exposure technics, and developing procedures must be ideal to obtain the correct radiographic results. X-ray beam angulation changes can distort the appearance of the crestal bone; overexposure can produce peripheral burnout of bone giving it an etched appearance; and developing technic errors can produce a film of high contrast which obliterates the fine bone trabeculae. For accurate evaluation of crestal bone height, the paralleling and bite-wing techniques are preferred to the bisecting the angle technique.

In periodontal disease, there may initially be widening of the periodontal ligament space at the crest of the proximal bone. Also, there may be localized erosion of the alveolar bone crest. Normally, the bone crest runs from the lamina dura of one tooth to that of the adjacent tooth and is flat and parallel to an imaginary line drawn from the cemento-enamel junctions of the two adjacent teeth. This normal interdental alveolar crestal bone has the same radiopacity as that of the lamina dura. In early periodontal disease, this alveolar crestal bone loses its radiopacity and becomes irregular and diffuse with a decreased radiographic density. The proximal crestal bone may, on occasions, show cupping. When the alveolar bone shows sclerosis between the lamina dura of two adjacent teeth, it must be looked upon favorably as a resistance to an irritant or reaction to occlusal stress.

In advanced periodontal disease one of the changes is the loss of crestal bone. Normally, the crestal bone is usually situated 1 to 2 mm apical to the cemento-enamel junction. When there is bone loss, the crestal bone is more than 2 mm apical to the cemento-enamel junction. Bone loss is considered horizontal when the crest of the proximal bone remains parallel to an imaginary line drawn between the cemento-enamel junctions of adjacent teeth. Horizontal bone loss may be localized or generalized. Generalized bone loss suggests a systemic etiology. Bone loss is considered vertical (angular) when the crest of the proximal bone is not parallel to the imaginary line drawn between the cemento-enamel junctions of adjacent teeth. Vertical bone loss is usually localized and related to such factors as trauma, calculus, subgingival plaque, overhanging restorations, and food impaction. In a multirooted tooth, bone loss involving the bifurcation (or trifurcation) of a root is called furcation involvement.

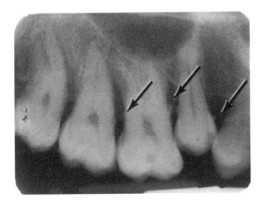

Figure 6–1

Calculus is prominently visible on the second premolar, first molar, and second molar. Calculus is visible on a radiograph only when it is sufficiently large in size. It is a contributing local factor to periodontal disease.

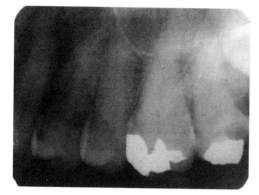

Figure 6–2

Effect of changes in horizonal angulation of the x-ray beam.

Figure A

Overlapping produced by incorrect horizontal angulation gives the illusion of the absence of calculus.

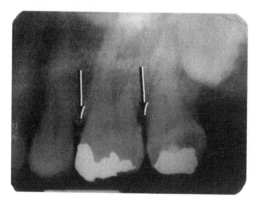

Figure B

Correct horizontal angulation shows the presence of calculus on the first molar and second premolar.

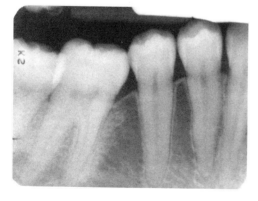

Figure 6–3

Normally, the crestal lamina dura extends to a point approximately 1 to 2 mm from the cemento-enamel junction. The bone crest running from the mesial of one tooth to the distal of the adjacent tooth normally appears flat and parallel to the imaginary line drawn from the cemento-enamel junctions of the same two teeth. This is clearly shown between the two premolars. The tilted first molar has slanted the mesial crestal bone but has maintained the parallelism. The normal alveolar crest, especially in a healthy condition, has an opacity not unlike that of the lamina dura.

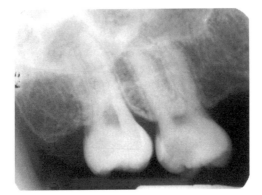

Figure 6–4

Over-eruption of the mesial molar has not disrupted the parallelism between the crestal bone and an imaginary line joining the cemento-enamel junctions of the two molars.

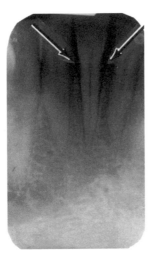

Figure 6–5

Widening of the periodontal ligament space at the crest of the proximal bone is observed on the mesial and distal proximals of the right central incisor. This may be indicative of occlusal trauma.

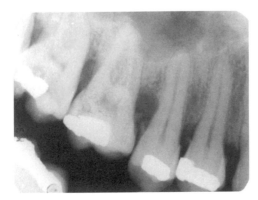

Figure 6–6

Resorption of alveolar crest is seen in several areas but is most prominent between the second premolar and first molar. Presence of large amount of calculus.

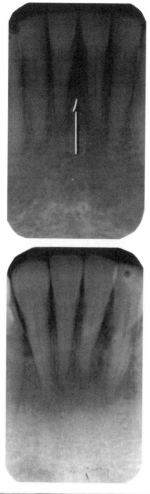

Figure 6–7

Cupping of alveolar crest inferior to the calculus between the two central incisors.

Figure 6–8

Crestal irregularities and destruction between the incisors in the presence of heavy calculus.

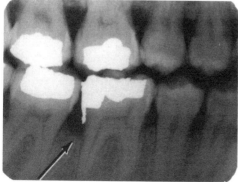

Figure 6–9

Overhang of amalgam restoration on distal of mandibular first molar is associated with loss of alveolar bone (arrow).

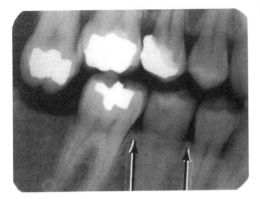

Figure 6–10
Effect of changes in vertical angulation (bite-wing and periapical radiographs).

Figure A
Bite-wing radiograph shows normal alveolar bone levels between the two mandibular premolars, and also between the mandibular second premolar and first molar.

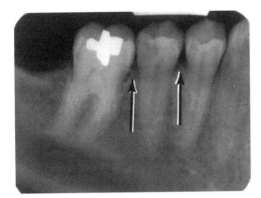

Figure B
Periapical radiograph made with excessive negative angulation of x-ray beam gives the illusion of bone growth between the mandibular premolars, and also between the second premolar and first molar.

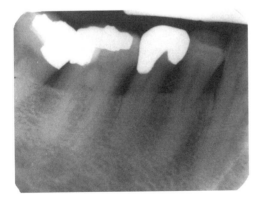

Figure 6–11
Horizontal bone loss proximal to the posterior teeth. Bone loss is considered horizontal when the crest of the proximal bone remains parallel to an imaginary line drawn between the cemento-enamel junctions of adjacent teeth.

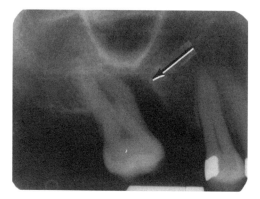

Figure 6–12

Vertical (angular) bone loss mesial to the maxillary molar. Bone loss is considered vertical when the crest of the proximal bone is not parallel to an imaginary line drawn between the cemento-enamel junctions of adjacent teeth.

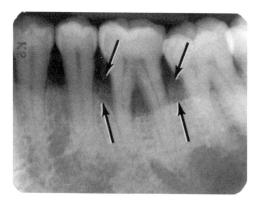

Figure 6–13

Superior arrows (pointing inferiorly) show the buccal bone level. Inferior arrows (pointing superiorly) show the lingual bone level.

The lingual bone level produces a sharp image because of its proximity to the film at the time of x-radiating the teeth. The buccal bone level produces a faint, unsharp image because of its distance from the film.

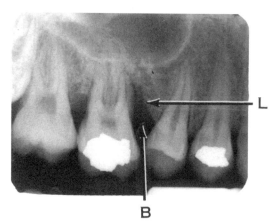

Figure 6–14

The proximal area between the second premolar and first molar shows vertical bone loss of the lingual bone (L) and horizontal bone loss of the buccal bone (B).

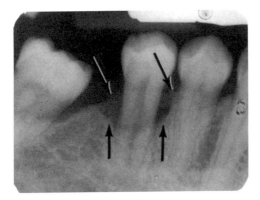

Figure 6–15

Buccal bone—superior arrows (pointing inferiorly) do not show any bone loss of the buccal plate.

Lingual bone—inferior arrows (pointing superiorly) show bone loss of the lingual plate.

Lingual bone level produces a sharp image because of its proximity to the film. Buccal bone level produces a faint, unsharp image because of its distance from the film.

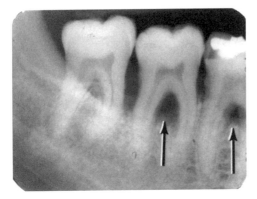

Figure 6–16

Furcation involvement of molar teeth in advanced periodontal disease.

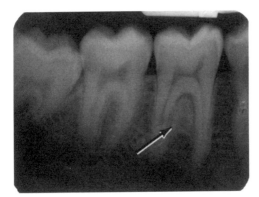

Figure 6–17

Bifurcation of the first molar shows sclerosis in the intraradicular bone.

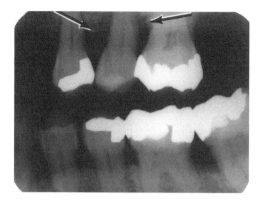

Figure 6–18

Effect of changes in vertical angulation (bite-wing and periapical radiographs).

Figure A

Bite-wing radiograph shows advanced bone loss between the maxillary teeth.

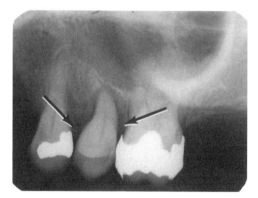

Figure B

Periapical radiograph made with excessive positive angulation of x-ray beam gives the illusion of bone growth between the maxillary teeth.

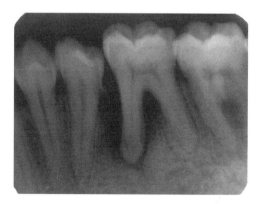

Figure 6–19

Dramatic loss of alveolar bone associated with the mesial root apex of the first molar in conjunction with a periodontal abscess.

JUVENILE PERIODONTITIS (PERIODONTOSIS) AND PAPILLON-LEFÈVRE SYNDROME

Juvenile periodontitis (periodontosis) is a type of rapidly progressing disease of the periodontium that typically arises in healthy adolescents and young adults. The disease is of obscure etiology and may have a hereditary component. Calculus may be absent since it is not an etiologic factor. Juvenile periodontitis may either be localized or generalized. The localized form involves only the first molars and incisors whereas the generalized form affects most of the dentition. Juvenile periodontitis is characterized by rapid alveolar bone loss in the presence of minimal plaque accumulation and clinical inflammation. The radiographic appearance is typically that of deep vertical (angular) bone loss with a marked predilection for the first molar and central incisor regions with relative sparing of other segments of the dentition. With excessive bone loss, the involved teeth loosen and become mobile. Treatment for juvenile periodontitis consists of scaling, root planing, curettage, and antibiotics. Osseous defects often respond to osseous grafts.

Papillon-Lefèvre Syndrome: This syndrome consists of

1) juvenile periodontitis (periodontosis);

2) palmar-plantar hyperkeratosis (hyperkeratosis of palms and soles);

3) hyperhidrosis (excessive sweating).

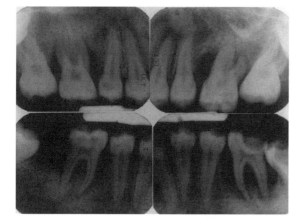

Figure 6–20A
Juvenile periodontitis (periodontosis). Notice the typical angular (vertical) bone loss and its typical location involving the first molars. Calculus is absent and is not an etiologic factor. The disease has a familial distribution.

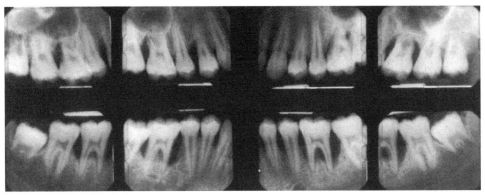

Figure 6–20B

Generalized juvenile periodontitis (periodontosis) shows typical deep vertical (angular) osseous defects affecting the maxillary and mandibular first molars as well as the premolars. This angular bone defect, especially involving the first molars, is characteristic of juvenile periodontitis.

DIABETES MELLITUS

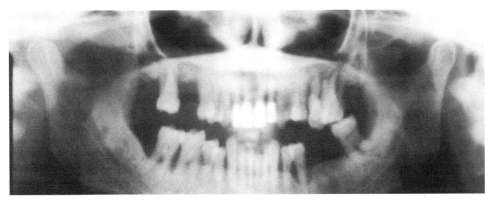

Figure 6–21

Uncontrolled diabetes mellitus (hypoinsulinism). There is marked bone loss and destruction of alveolar bone. Uncontrolled diabetes mellitus in itself does not cause periodontal disease; however, it tends to increase the incidence and severity of periodontal disease. Also see Chapter 18 (Genetic and Metabolic Diseases).

SCLERODERMA

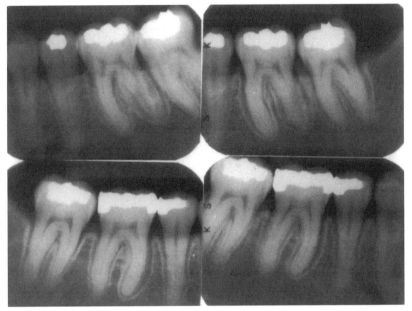

Figure 6–22

Scleroderma. There is widening of the periodontal ligament space around several teeth. The lamina dura around the affected teeth remains intact and uninvolved. Clinically, scleroderma causes sclerosis of the skin and of other tissues.

HISTIOCYTOSIS X

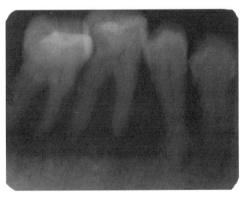

Figure 6–23

Histiocytosis X has caused complete destruction of the interdental alveolar bone in the molar region. Described as floating teeth. Also see Chapter 15 (Nonodontogenic Benign Tumors of the Jaws).

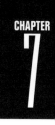

APICAL
LESIONS

Periapical granuloma

Radicular cyst

Apical abscess

Apical scar

Surgical defect

Periodontal disease

Condensing osteitis

Osteosclerosis

Socket sclerosis

Periapical cemental dysplasia

Cementifying fibroma (ossifying fibroma)

Cementoblastoma

Florid osseous dysplasia

APICAL LESIONS

Whenever a lesion is observed on a radiograph, it must first be described in general terms before a differential diagnosis is attempted. Is the lesion radiolucent, radiopaque, or mixed (combination of radiolucency and radiopacity)? Where is the lesion located? The apices of which teeth are involved? What is the size of the lesion? Is the margin of the lesion ill-defined, well-defined, or well-defined with a radiopaque border? Is the appearance of the bone surrounding the lesion normal, porous, or sclerotic?

The various radiographic appearances of the margins of lesions and the changes in the surrounding bone have been given clinical interpretation by some diagnosticians based largely on intuitive analysis rather than on research data. Although the significance of these signs is sometimes questionable, they are useful in radiographic interpretation. An ill-defined (diffuse, irregular) periphery is suggestive of a lesion enlarging by invading the surrounding bone. A well-defined (circumscribed) periphery is suggestive of a self-contained lesion enlarging by expansion. A well-defined periphery with a hyperostotic (sclerotic) radiopaque periphery is suggestive of an extremely slow-growing, self-contained lesion enlarging by expansion.

If the bone surrounding a lesion does not show any change, the clinical interpretation is that of a static lesion. If it shows porosity (destructive breakdown), the interpretation is that of an invasive process resulting from osteolytic activity. If it shows sclerosis (hyperostosis), the interpretation is that of resistance to the pathologic process resulting from osteoblastic activity.

TYPES OF BORDERS

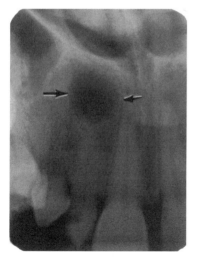

Figure 7–1
Well-defined radiolucent lesion at the apex of the maxillary lateral incisor. The circumscribed radiopaque (sclerotic) border signifies that the lesion is self-contained, enlarges by expansion, and is slow-growing. There is no change in the surrounding bone.

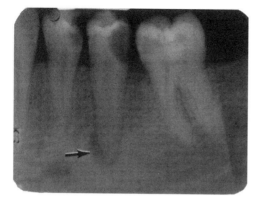

Figure 7–2

Well-defined radiolucent lesion at the apex of the mandibular left second premolar. The well-defined border signifies that the lesion is self-contained and enlarges by expansion. The surrounding bone shows slight sclerosis (osteoblastic activity) which signifies resistance to the pathologic process.

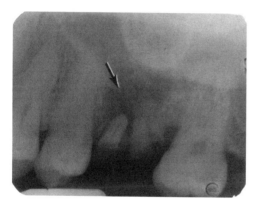

Figure 7–3

A radiolucent lesion with diffuse, irregular borders at the apices of the roots of the maxillary left first molar. The diffuse margins and the porosity (osteolytic activity) in surrounding bone signify an invasive process.

PERIODONTAL SPACE WIDENING (APICAL PERIODONTITIS)

Radiographically, apparent widening (also called thickening) of the periodontal ligament space is caused by edema, resulting in accumulation of inflammatory exudate in the connective tissue of the periodontal ligament. The term apical periodontitis is often used to describe this pathologic periodontal space widening.

Pathologic periodontal space widening occurs as a result of infection, trauma, orthodontic treatment, or tooth extrusion. It is imperative that dentists be aware of trauma resulting from occlusal imbalance, especially that caused by an amalgam, gold, composite resin, or other restoration that is placed too high in the tooth and results in premature contact with the opposing tooth. Depending on the extent of the traumatic force and the individual's physiologic resistance, the widened periodontal space either returns to its normal appearance after the elimination of the trauma or may form a chronic apical inflammatory lesion such as an apical granuloma, a radicular cyst, or an apical abscess.

Nonpathologic periodontal space widening occurs as a result of the terminal stage of root formation (dental papilla), wide marrow space superimposed on a tooth apex, or superimposition of a tooth apex on a radiolucent anatomy (such as a nasal fossa, maxillary sinus, mental foramen or submandibular fossa) producing overexposure or burnout. An illusion of loss of lamina dura may also be produced when a tooth apex is superimposed on a radiolucent anatomy.

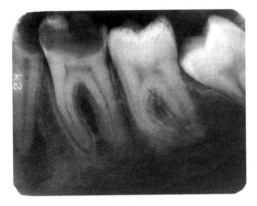

Figure 7–4

Infection (caries) is the cause of the widened periodontal space of the first molar (apical periodontitis). In this case, the lamina dura is also thickened (radiopaque line).

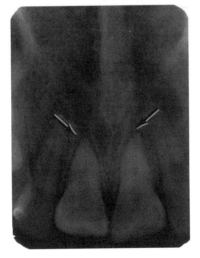

Figure 7–5

Trauma is the cause of the widened periodontal spaces of the central incisors (apical periodontitis). Clinically, the teeth were retruded.

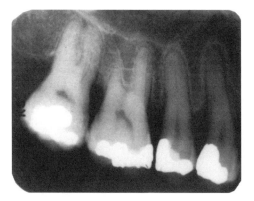

Figure 7–6

Traumatic occlusion, that is, premature contact with the opposing premolars, is the cause of the widened periodontal spaces of the maxillary premolars (apical periodontitis). The patient also has alveolar bone loss due to periodontal disease.

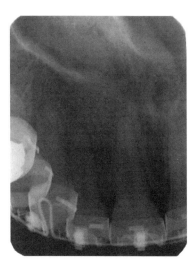

Figure 7–7

Orthodontic treatment is the cause of the widened periodontal spaces of the incisors. After completion of treatment, the periodontal spaces return to their normal appearances.

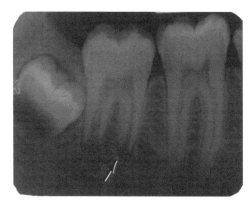

Figure 7–8

Developing root apices of the second molar may be mistaken for widened periodontal spaces. Root apices complete their formation approximately one to two years after tooth eruption.

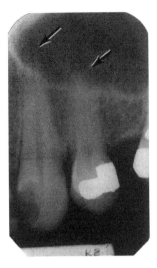

Figure 7–9

Illusion of widened periodontal space of the root apex of the premolar because of superimposition on a radiolucent anatomy (maxillary sinus). The widened periodontal space of the canine may be due to a similar illusion and/or infection (caries). Also note the illusion of loss of apical lamina dura on both teeth.

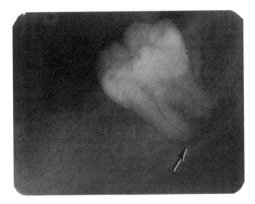

Figure 7–10

Illusion of widened periodontal spaces of the root apices of the molar because of superimposition on a radiolucent anatomy (mandibular canal). Also note the illusion of apical loss of lamina dura.

APICAL LESION VERSUS ANATOMICAL LANDMARK

To differentiate an apical lesion from an anatomical landmark, make another radiograph with a different x-ray beam angulation. An anatomical landmark will change its position with a change in angulation of the x-ray beam. On the other hand, an apical lesion will maintain the same relationship to the involved tooth. (See Figs. 1–73A and 1–73B).

Another method of differentiation is to follow the continuity of the periodontal space. The periodontal space will be interrupted in the case of an apical lesion but will be continuous in the case of an anatomical landmark.

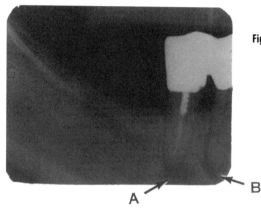

Figure 7–11
A—Mental foramen. Notice the intact periodontal space.
B—Chronic inflammatory apical lesion. Notice the loss of the apical periodontal space.

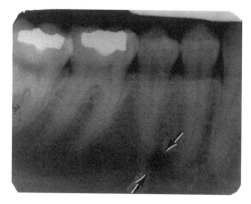

Figure 7–12
Radiolucent anatomy mistaken for an apical lesion. Mental foramen superimposed on the root apex of the second premolar may be mistaken for an apical lesion.

PERIAPICAL GRANULOMA, RADICULAR CYST AND APICAL ABSCESS (INFLAMMATORY PULPO-PERIAPICAL LESIONS)

The most common pathologic conditions that involve teeth are the inflammatory lesions of the pulp and periapical areas. Once inflammation (pulpitis) has spread from the dental pulp, it can produce a variety of apical pathologic changes, the most common of which are the periapical granuloma, radicular cyst, and apical abscess. Various factors such as the host's resistance and the virulence of the bacteria affect the local inflammatory response in the periapical area. Without a microscopic diagnosis, a clinician is frequently unable to differentiate between a periapical granuloma, a radicular cyst, and an apical abscess. Radiographic examination is inadequate in making a specific diagnosis.

Inflammatory periapical lesions have the following common clinical characteristics:

1. A history of painful pulpitis leading to the death of the pulp;

2. A nonvital reaction to electric pulp testing. In a multirooted tooth where only one root is associated with the pulpo-periapical pathosis, the tooth will frequently give a vital reaction;

3. Presence of a deep carious lesion exposing the pulp or a restoration close to the pulp, or a fractured tooth and/or a discolored crown;

4. Destruction resulting in an interrupted lamina dura of the involved tooth.

A **granuloma** is formed from the successful attempt of the periapical tissues to neutralize and confine the irritating toxic products escaping from the root canal. This low grade inflammation in the tissues continues to induce the proliferation of vascular granulation tissue. A granuloma may evolve into a radicular cyst or an apical abscess. Clinically, the lesion is usually asymptomatic but may sometimes exhibit mild pain and sensitivity to percussion. The affected tooth is nonvital. Radiographically, granulomas form small well-defined radiolucencies. They are the most common periapical lesions and constitute approximately 50 percent of all periapical radiolucent lesions.

A **radicular cyst** (also known as periapical cyst, dental cyst, periodontal cyst) has its origin from the cell rests of Malassez which are present in periodontal and periapical ligament, and in periapical granulomas. Most radicular cysts originate from pre-existing granulomas. Clinically, the lesion is usually asymptomatic but may sometimes exhibit mild pain and sensitivity to percussion. The affected tooth is nonvital. A radicular cyst may slowly enlarge and when large, may cause expansion of the cortical plates. Radiographically, a radicular cyst forms a large well-defined radiolucency with or without a radiopaque (hyperostotic) border. The more pronounced the hyperostotic (sclerotic) border, the more likely is the lesion to be a radicular cyst. It is the second most common periapical lesion and constitutes approximately 40 percent of all periapical radiolucent lesions. (See also Chapter 12, Cysts of the Jaws).

In approximately 90 percent of the cases, a well-defined radiolucency at the apex of an untreated asymptomatic tooth with a nonvital or diseased pulp is either a dental granuloma or a radicular cyst. Their sizes are the differentiating features: a granuloma is small whereas a radicular cyst is large. In practice, however, it is not necessary to differentiate a periapical granuloma from a radicular cyst because both lesions respond quite well to conservative root canal therapy.

An **apical abscess,** also called dental or dentoalveolar abscess, usually develops from a pulpo-periapical inflammatory condition. In the acute stage, the onset of infection is so sudden that there is no radiographic evidence of an apical lesion. An apical abscess can develop also from a pre-existing granuloma or cyst. The associated tooth is nonvital, very painful, extremely sensitive to percussion, and often slightly extruded. The patient will complain that the tooth position feels high when it occludes with the opposing tooth. The tooth will not respond to electrical pulp tests. The application of ice will slightly relieve the pain but the application of heat will intensify pain. The tooth may demonstrate increased mobility. Radiographically, apical abscesses form large radiolucencies with diffuse irregular borders. They are the least common of the three pulpo-periapical lesions and constitute approximately 2 percent of all periapical radiolucent lesions.

If an apical abscess is permitted to progress without treatment, it may penetrate the cortical plate at the thinnest and closest part of the tooth apex and form a swelling in the adjacent soft tissues. This infection site in the soft tissues is painful. The skin or mucous surface over the abscess is warm and rubbery to palpation, and demonstrates fluctuance. Once drainage is established by a sinus tract permitting the pus to drain to the surface, the tooth and associated swelling are no longer painful since the pain-producing pressure of the abscess is reduced. The regional lymph nodes may be enlarged and painful. The systemic temperature may be elevated.

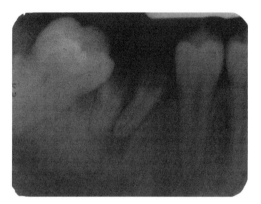

Figure 7–13
   Presence of either a periapical granuloma, a radicular cyst or an abscess at the root apices of the first molar. The small, well-defined radiolucency is suggestive (on a speculative basis) of a periapical granuloma. Periapical granulomas are the most frequently occurring of the three inflammatory periapical lesions. The involved tooth is nonvital.

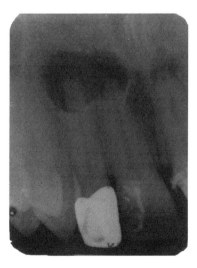

Figure 7–14
   Presence of either a periapical granuloma, a radicular cyst or an abscess at the root apices of the right central and lateral incisors. The large, well-defined radiolucency with a radiopaque (sclerotic) border is suggestive (on a speculative basis) of a radicular cyst (periapical cyst). Radicular cysts are the second most frequently occurring of the three inflammatory periapical lesions. The involved tooth is nonvital.

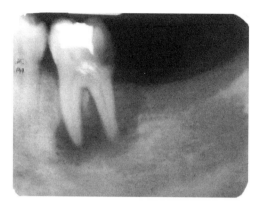

Figure 7–15

Presence of either a periapical granuloma, a radicular cyst or an abscess at the root apices of the first molar. The large radiolucency with diffuse irregular border is suggestive (on a speculative basis) of an abscess. Apical abscesses are the least frequently occurring of the three inflammatory periapical lesions. The involved tooth is nonvital.

APICAL SCAR

An inflammatory apical lesion treated by root canal therapy may respond well to treatment by filling new bone at the site of the lesion. However, the healing process may sometimes terminate abruptly and leave a small amount of dense scar tissue known as an apical scar. The scar tissue represents one of the possible end points of healing. It is composed of dense fibrous tissue and is situated at the apex of a pulpless tooth in which the root canals have been successfully filled. Microscopic examination reveals fibroblasts scattered in the collagen fibers. Unlike an apical granuloma, inflammatory cells are not a feature and vascularity is quite meager. An apical scar is a small, asymptomatic, and well-circumscribed radiolucency. When observed radiographically over the years, it will either remain constant in size or diminish slightly.

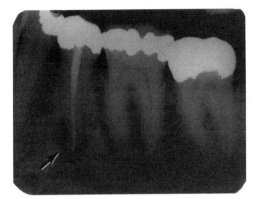

Figure 7–16

Apical scar is an area at the apex of a tooth that fails to fill in with osseous tissue after endodontic treatment. The second premolar was successfully treated with root canal therapy. The apical radiolucency persisted after treatment. Patient was recalled after several months. The radiolucency slightly decreased in size but was still present.

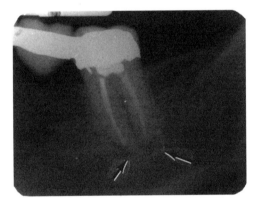

Figure 7–17

Apical scar. The molar was successfully treated with root canal therapy. Patient was recalled after several months. The apical radiolucency reduced in size and persisted.

SURGICAL DEFECT

A surgical defect is that portion of bone that fails to form osseous tissue. It is frequently seen periapically after root resection when the site is filled with dense fibrous (collagen) tissue instead of bone. It is an asymptomatic persistent radiolucency. An extraction site can also form a surgical defect. Approximately 75 percent of all surgically treated periapical radiolucencies require 1 to 10 years or longer for complete resolution. In the remaining 25 percent, complete healing does not occur.

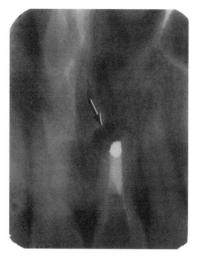

Figure 7–18

Surgical defect in bone is an area that fails to fill in with osseous tissue after surgery. An apicoectomy was performed at the apex of the left central incisor and the lesion was curetted. The radiolucency persisted as a surgical defect.

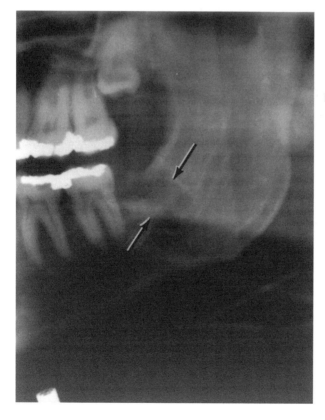

Figure 7–19

Surgical defect at the extraction site of the mandibular third molar. The radiolucency of the tooth socket persisted after one year.

PERIODONTAL DISEASE

Periodontal disease is discussed in detail in a previous chapter. Nevertheless, it is considered here because it produces a relatively common periapical radiolucency in the advanced stages. The entire bony support of the involved tooth may be completely destroyed or the tooth may appear to be floating in a radiolucency. Sometimes a narrow vertical pocket may extend to the apex and appear as a well-defined periapical radiolucency. This may lead the unwary clinician to a false conclusion of a pulpo-periapical pathosis. In the advanced stages, these teeth are usually quite mobile and may become sensitive to percussion; but surprisingly, many remain vital, and the demonstration of such vitality aids the clinician in differentiating a periodontal disease radiolucency from an inflammatory apical radiolucency (periapical granuloma, radicular cyst and apical abscess). A clinical examination of supporting tooth structures should be undertaken by probing all periodontal pockets.

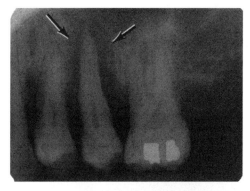

Figure 7–20
Periodontal disease producing a periapical radiolucency. Vertical bone loss around the second premolar extends to the apex and appears as a fairly well-defined radiolucency. The affected tooth is vital.

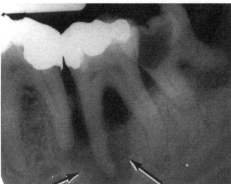

Figure 7–21
Periodontal disease producing a periapical radiolucency around the mesial root of the second molar. Vertical bone loss extends to the apex of the root. The affected tooth is vital.

CONDENSING OSTEITIS
(FOCAL SCLEROSING OSTEOMYELITIS)

Condensing osteitis is a reaction of bone induced by inflammation. It occurs mainly at the apex of a tooth from an infected pulp. The infection from tooth caries reaches the pulp and progresses to the apical tissues to produce a small periapical radiolucency called rarefying osteitis. The small rarefying osteitis may be either a periapical granuloma, a radicular cyst or an abscess. The bone surrounding this rarefying osteitis becomes dense in order to prevent further spread of the lesion. This dense radiopacity surrounding the rarefying osteitis is called condensing osteitis. The pulp of the involved tooth is nonvital.

1. Condensing osteitis is a reaction to periapical infection resulting in the formation of dense bone. The infection usually originates from caries (sometimes from periodontal disease).

2. Condensing osteitis occurs usually at the apex of a nonvital tooth. On a radiograph, the tooth may exhibit a large carious lesion or a large restoration close to the dental pulp.

3. Radiographically, the lesion shows a diffuse radiopacity surrounding a small central radiolucency at the apex (or apices) of a tooth.

4. Treatment consists of removing the infection either through tooth extraction or root canal therapy.

5. Prognosis—the high radiopacity of bone tends to disappear partially or completely in a majority of cases after treatment is given to remove the infection. Approximately 30 percent of the cases will not resolve to normal appearing bone after adequate treatment. The persistence of the radiopacity should not be of concern to the clinician because of the innocuous nature of the lesion.

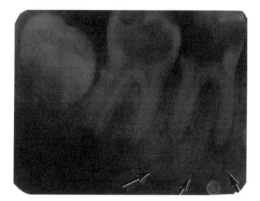

Figure 7–22

Condensing osteitis at the root apices of the carious first molar. Condensing osteitis is a reaction to an inflammatory process. Note the diffuse radiopacities (condensing osteitis) surrounding the apical radiolucencies (rarefying osteitis). The involved tooth is nonvital.

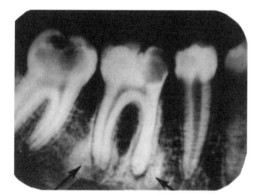

Figure 7–23

Condensing osteitis at the root apices of the carious first molar. Note the diffuse radiopacities (condensing osteitis) surrounding the apical radiolucencies (rarefying osteitis). The involved tooth is nonvital.

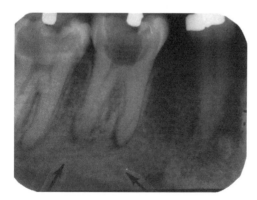

Figure 7–24

Condensing osteitis at the root apices of the carious first and second molars. The involved teeth are nonvital.

OSTEOSCLEROSIS AND SOCKET SCLEROSIS

Osteosclerosis (enostosis) is one of the common bony lesions found incidentally on a radiographic examination. It is a well-defined radiopaque mass without any associated radiolucency. The cause of the lesion is not known (idiopathic). The lesion is asymptomatic and the teeth associated with it are invariably healthy with vital pulps. There is neither any pain nor any cortical bone expansion. The lesion may occur either in the alveolus, in the periapical region, in the intra-radicular or inter-radicular region, below the crest of the ridge, or in the body of the mandible.

It has been suggested that excess occlusal stress may be one of the factors in osteosclerosis associated with roots of teeth. When it occurs near the first and second premolars, its formation is speculated to be that of deposition of sclerotic bone around the root fragment of a deciduous molar which acts as a nidus. It has been reported that only 10% to 12% of patients with osteosclerosis show root resorption of an adjoining tooth.

When osteosclerosis occurs in the socket of an extracted tooth as a reparative process, it is known as socket sclerosis. Radiographically, it is often impossible to distinguish socket sclerosis from a retained root of a tooth. A dentist may be wrongfully accused of having failed to remove the tooth in its entirety.

1. Osteosclerosis refers to a localized region of abnormally dense bone. The cause of the sclerotic bone is either idiopathic or reparative. It is not associated with any infection.

2. Osteosclerosis can occur in any part of the jaw, even at the apices of vital teeth. Socket sclerosis occurs in the sockets of extracted teeth and may sometimes be mistaken for retained roots.

3. Radiographically, the lesion shows a well-defined radiopacity. There is no association with any radiolucency. Ten to twelve percent of patients show root resorption.

4. No treatment is necessary.

5. Prognosis—the radiopacity persists without any increase in size.

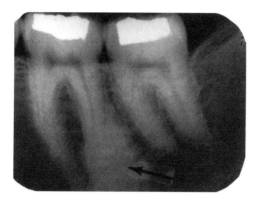

Figure 7–25
Osteosclerosis at the root apices of the first molar. The involved tooth is vital.

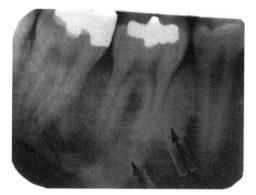

Figure 7–26
Osteosclerosis between the second premolar and first molar, and at the mesial root apex of the first molar. The involved tooth is vital. Ten to twelve percent of the patients show root resorption.

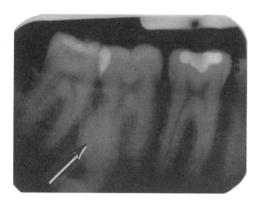

Figure 7–27
Osteosclerosis at the distal root of the second molar.

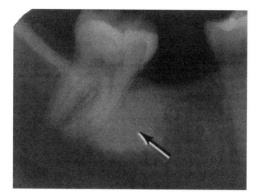

Figure 7–28

Osteosclerotic bone to the mesial of the molar, preventing the tooth from further tilting or drifting.

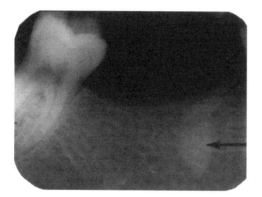

Figure 7–29

Socket sclerosis. Sclerosing bone deposited in the socket of the extracted tooth. A dentist may be erroneously accused of having failed to extract the root. There are no definite radiographic criteria for distinguishing a retained root from a socket sclerosis.

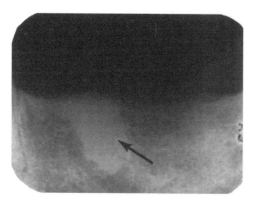

Figure 7–30

Socket sclerosis. Although there are no definite radiographic criteria for distinguishing a retained root from a socket sclerosis, in this case, the diffuse border distinguishes socket sclerosis from a retained root.

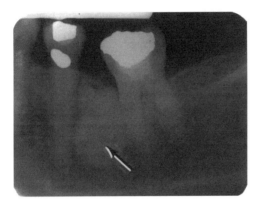

Figure 7–31
Socket sclerosis between the second premolar and the mesially drifted second molar.

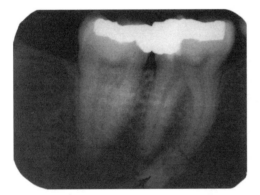

Figure 7–32
Osteosclerosis around the walls of the nutrient canal at the apex of the mesial root of the first molar. A nutrient canal wall acts as a nidus for deposition of sclerotic bone. The involved tooth is vital.

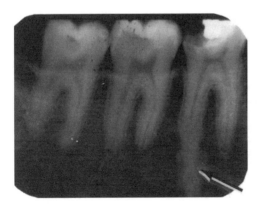

Figure 7–33
Osteosclerosis around the walls of the nutrient canal at the distal root apex of the first molar A nutrient canal wall acts as a nidus for deposition of sclerotic bone. The involved tooth is vital.

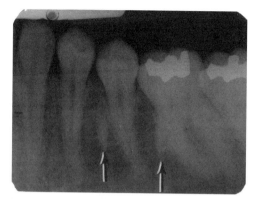

Figure 7–34

Retained root tips of deciduous second molar. It is hypothesized that a retained deciduous root tip acts as a nidus for osteosclerosis.

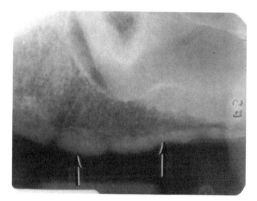

Figure 7–35

Hyperostosis is osteosclerotic bone that appears on the crest of the alveolar ridge.

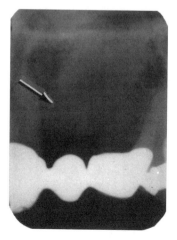

Figure 7–36

Hyperostosis beneath a bridge pontic.

CEMENTOMAS

A. Periapical cemental dysplasia (periapical cementoma, apical cementoma)

B. Cementifying fibroma (ossifying fibroma, cemento-ossifying fibroma)

C. Cementoblastoma (true cementoma)

Periapical cemental dysplasia, cementifying fibroma, ossifying fibroma, cemento-ossifying fibroma, cementoblastoma, and florid osseous dysplasia have been grouped by some under the term "benign fibro-osseous lesions of periodontal ligament origin." These benign fibro-osseous lesions of periodontal ligament origin are a group of cementum- and bone-producing tumors and tumor-like proliferations that arise from the cells of the periodontal ligament. In this text, the florid osseous dysplasia is described as a separate entity.

All the three types of cementomas have three radiographic appearances which follow:

1. Early or osteolytic stage appears radiolucent

2. Mixed or cementoblastic stage appears as a radiolucency containing radiopacities

3. Final or calcified stage appears as a homogeneous radiopacity surrounded by a thin radiolucent border.

All cementomas are associated with teeth having vital pulps, unless otherwise involved with caries or trauma. See also Chapter 14 (Odontogenic Begnign Tumors of the Jaws).

PERIAPICAL CEMENTAL DYSPLASIA

Black persons and females of 40 years and older are more commonly affected than white persons and males with periapical cemental dysplasia. Although periapical cemental dysplasia occurs usually in the mandibular anterior region, it may sometimes be found in the mandibular posterior region. On a radiograph, the early radiolucent stage of periapical cemental dysplasia could be misdiagnosed for inflammatory periapical radiolucencies (periapical granuloma, radicular cyst, abscess). An unalert clinician might needlessly extract or institute endodontic treatment on a tooth with a normal pulp. The periapical cemental dysplasia is associated with a vital tooth and is totally asymptomatic. These features are in contrast to those of an inflammatory lesion which is associated with a nonvital tooth and may exhibit symptoms.

Periapical Cemental Dysplasia (Periapical cementoma)	*Cementifying Fibroma (Ossifying fibroma, cemento-ossifying fibroma)	*Cementoblastoma (True cementoma)
1. Believed to be a reaction of periapical bone. Actual cause unknown. Asymptomatic.	Benign mesenchymal odontogenic neoplasm.	Benign mesenchymal odontogenic neoplasm.
2. Average age is 40 years. Predominantly in black persons and in females.	In young and middle-aged adults.	In teenagers and young adults.
3. Around apices of teeth. Usually mandibular anteriors.	Around apices of teeth. Usually the mandibular posteriors.	Attached to the apex or apices of mandibular molar or premolar.
4. Vital teeth. Position of teeth not affected.	Vital teeth. Displacement of teeth or divergence of roots.	Vital teeth. Position of teeth not affected.
5. Usually multilocular. Sometimes unilocular.	Usually unilocular.	Usually unilocular.
6. Radiographic appearance has three developmental stages.	Radiographic appearance has three developmental stages.	Radiographic appearance when discovered is usually of the third stage.
7. No expansion of cortical plates. Self-limiting lesion.	Expansion of cortical plates.	Expansion of cortical plates when large.
8. No treatment necessary.	Excision of lesion.	Extraction of involved tooth and excision of lesion.

*See also Chapter 14, Odontogenic Benign Tumors of the Jaws.

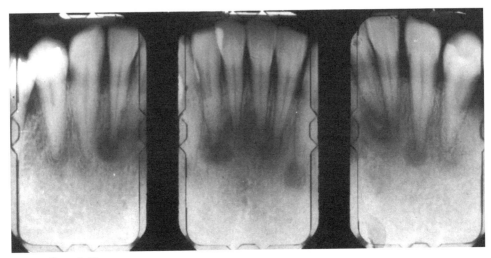

Figure 7–37

Periapical cemental dysplasia (early stage). Multiple radiolucencies at the apices of the mandibular anterior teeth. In periapical cemental dysplasia, the teeth are vital unless otherwise involved with caries or trauma. The radiolucencies should not be misdiagnosed as inflammatory apical lesions (granulomas, cysts, abscess) in which the teeth are nonvital and may be symptomatic.

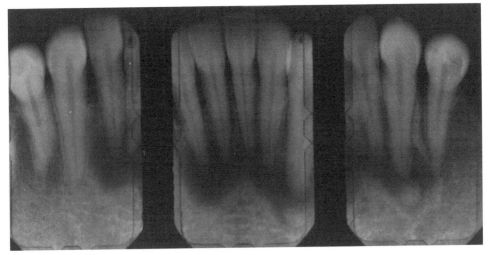

Figure 7–38

Periapical cemental dysplasia (early stage). Unilocular large radiolucency at the apices of vital mandibular anterior teeth. The radiolucency should not be misdiagnosed as an inflammatory apical lesion. In periapical cemental dysplasia, the teeth are vital and totally asymptomatic.

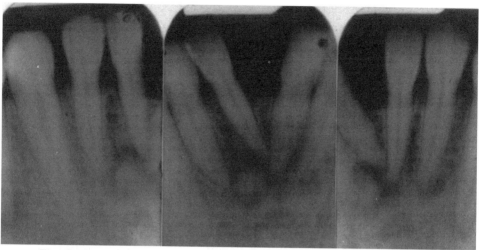

Figure 7–39

Periapical cemental dysplasia (mixed stage). Multiple radiolucencies containing faint opacifications at the apices of the mandibular anterior teeth.

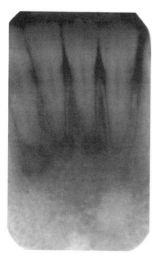

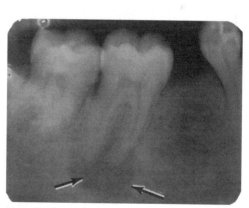

Figure 7–40

Periapical cemental dysplasia (calcified stage). Each radiopacity is surrounded by a radiolucent border at the apices of mandibular incisor teeth.

Figure 7–41

Cementoblastoma (early stage). Unilocular circular radiolucency at the apices of the mandibular first molar. The involved tooth is vital. See also Chapter 14 (Odontogenic Benign Tumors of the Jaws).

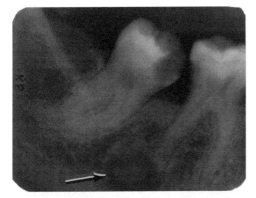

Figure 7–42

Cementoblastoma (mixed stage). Unilocular circular radiolucency containing faint opacification. The involved tooth is vital. See also Chapter 14 (Odontogenic Benign Tumors of the Jaws).

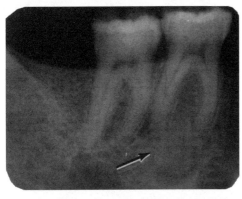

Figure 7–43

Cementoblastoma (calcified stage). A dense circular radiopacity surrounded by a radiolucent border at the apices of the mandibular first molar. A cementoblastoma is usually discovered radiographically in the calcified stage.

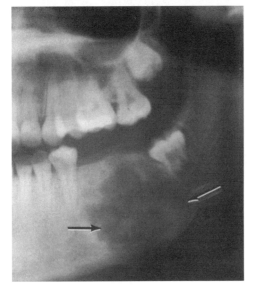

Figure 7–44

Cementifying fibroma or ossifying fibroma (osteolytic stage) in the mandibular first and second molar region. Unilocular radiolucency containing faint opacification. Well-defined cortical margins. See also Chapter 14 (Odontogenic Benign Tumors of the Jaws).

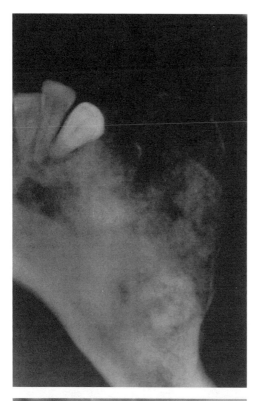

Figure 7–45

Cementifying or ossifying fibroma (calcified stage). Occlusal view shows buccal expansion of the mixed radiopaque-radiolucent lesion. See also Chapter 14 (Odontogenic Benign Tumors of the Jaws).

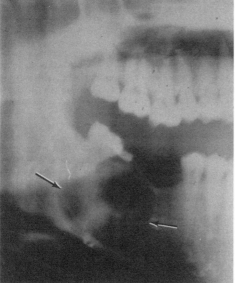

Figure 7–46

Cemento-ossifying fibroma (mixed stage). The large unilocular radiolucency containing calcifications shows expansion of the cortical plate near the inferior border of the mandible.

FLORID OSSEOUS DYSPLASIA (DIFFUSE CEMENTOSIS, CHRONIC DIFFUSE SCLEROSING OSTEOMYELITIS, GIGANTIFORM CEMENTOMAS, MULTIPLE ENOSTOSES, CHRONIC SCLEROSING CEMENTOSIS)

Florid osseous dysplasia, also known as chronic diffuse sclerosing osteomyelitis, is a reactive type of fibro-osseous bone disease with a marked predilection for black, middle-aged females of 40 years and older. Some pathologists consider this bony dysplastic lesion as an exuberant form of periapical cemental dysplasia. Mandibular involvement is more common than maxillary involvement. The teeth are vital unless otherwise involved with caries or trauma. The lesion consists of multiple dense radiopacities surrounded by narrow peripheral radiolucent rims. These radiopacities are symmetrically distributed in two or all four jaw quadrants. The coalescing radiopaque masses may sometimes obscure the peripheral radiolucent rims, resulting in diffuse radiopacities without any associated radiolucency. Usually there is no jaw expansion and is discovered incidentally during radiographic examination. Sometimes, advanced cases may show a painless expansion of the alveolar process, necessitating the need to adjust dentures. The lesion is restricted to the jawbones and must be differentiated from generalized conditions like Paget's disease and osteopetrosis. Tooth extraction in the affected area exposes the avascular cementum to the oral cavity. This avascular cementum is prone to infection and may lead to chronic suppurative osteomyelitis with draining fistulous tracts.

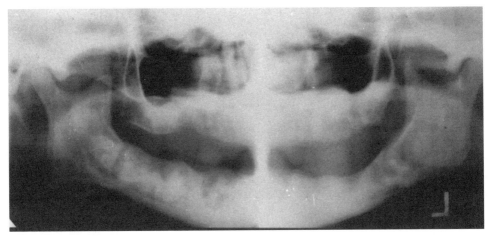

Figure 7–47
Florid osseous dysplasia. Diffuse opaque masses with radiolucent borders involving both sides of the mandible.

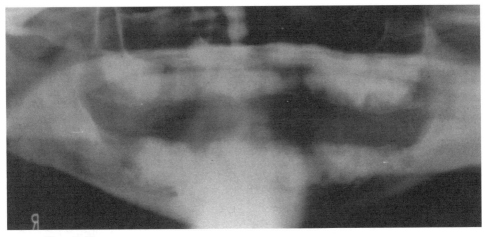

Figure 7–48
Florid osseous dysplasia (also known as chronic diffuse sclerosing osteomyelitis). Pagetoid cotton-wool appearance with diffuse, irregularly shaped radiopaque areas without any associated radiolucency and involving all four quadrants of the jaws.

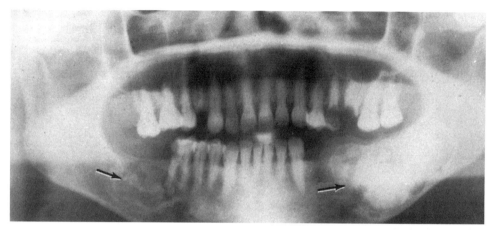

Figure 7–49

Florid osseous dysplasia. Bilaterally located in the mandible, well-circumscribed, radiopaque masses surrounded by radiolucencies. In florid osseous dysplasia, the teeth are vital unless otherwise involved with caries or trauma.

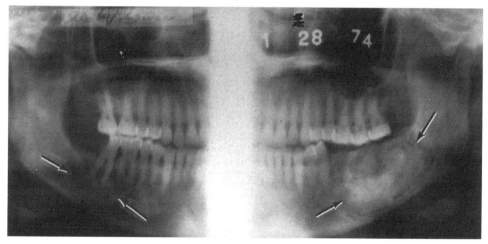

Figure 7–50

Florid osseous dysplasia. Bilaterally located radiopaque masses surrounded by peripheral radiolucent borders similar to those of periapical cemental dysplasia.

MEDULLARY SPACES, AND TORI

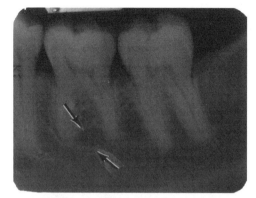

Figure 7–51

Large medullary space (large marrow space, wide inter-trabecular space) between the roots of the first molar. May be misdiagnosed as an apical lesion.

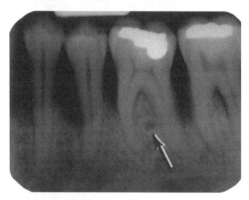

Figure 7–52

Large medullary spaces (large marrow spaces, wide inter-trabecular spaces) between the roots of the first molar. May be misdiagnosed as a lesion.

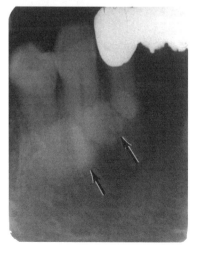

Figure 7–53

Mandibular tori superimposed on the roots of the lateral incisor, canine and first premolar.

133

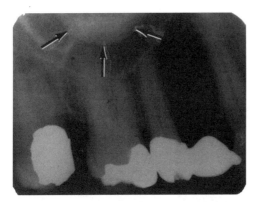

Figure 7–54
Torus palatinus (palatal torus).

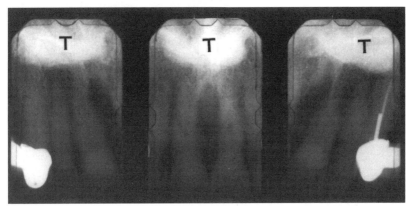

Figure 7–55
Torus palatinus (T) as seen on anterior films. May be misdiagnosed as osteosclerosis.

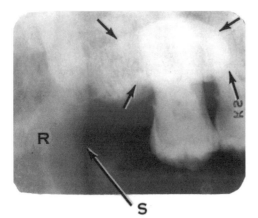

Figure 7–56
Four small arrows—Exostosis evident on buccal surface of alveolar ridge. Exostoses are similar to torus palatinus and mandibular tori but are located on the buccal aspect of the alveolus.

R—Ramus of mandible

S—Anterior border of ramus

PERIAPICAL RADIOLUCENCIES

Granuloma

Radicular Cyst

Abscess

Apical scar

Surgical defect

Periodontal disease

Cementomas (osteolytic stage)

Chronic suppurative osteomyelitis (See also Chapter 13
   Osteomyelitis).

PERIAPICAL RADIOPACITIES

Cementomas (calcified stage)

Condensing osteitis

Osteosclerosis

Socket sclerosis

Florid osseous dysplasia (diffuse cementosis)

Tori

Hypercementosis

TECHNIQUE ERRORS AND ARTIFACTS

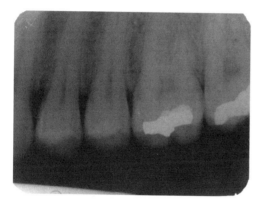

Figure 8–1

The root apices of the premolars and molars are cut off because the film was placed too closely to the teeth in the maxillary arch when using the paralleling technique.

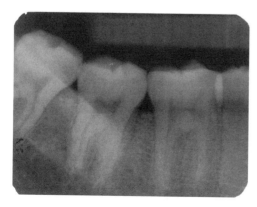

Figure 8–2

Radiograph of the mandibular molar region does not show all of the specific region on the film. The third molar has been cut off. The film needs to be placed more posteriorly.

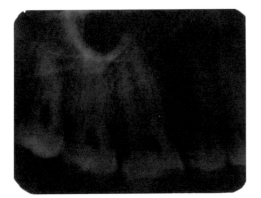

Figure 8–3

High film density. The dark radiograph is due to an error either in exposure factors, in processing factors, or in patient characteristics.

1. Exposure errors include high mA, high kVp, high exposure time, or short source-film distance.
2. Processing errors include fogged film; high developing temperature; films left in developer for longer than usual time; depleted, contaminated or exhausted solutions;
3. Patient characteristics include x-raying edentulous, pediatric, or small-face patients without a corresponding reduction in any one of the exposure factors (mA, kVp, or time).

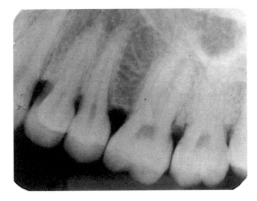

Figure 8–4

Low film density. The light radiograph is due to an error in exposure factors, in processing factors, or in patient characteristics.

1. Exposure errors include low mA, low kVp, low exposure time, or long source-film distance.
2. Processing errors include low developing temperature, films left in developer for shorter than usual time, dilute solutions, or films left in fixer for an extended period of time.
3. Patient characteristics include x-raying big-face or dense-bone patients without a corresponding increase in any one of the exposure factors (mA,kVp, or time). (Low film density due to herringbone, tire-track, or honeycomb effect is discussed separately because of its characteristic radiographic appearance See Figs. 8–20 and 8–21).

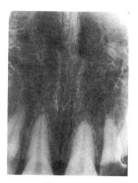
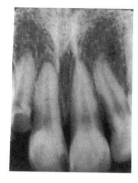
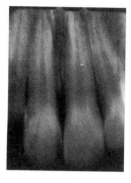

Figure 8–5

Incorrect vertical angulation produces shape distortion in bisecting the angle technique: (left) foreshortening due to overangulation; that is, increased vertical angulation of cone (PID) in relation to the occlusal plane; (center) correct length of teeth without any distortion; (right) elongation due to underangulation; that is, decreased vertical angulation in relation to the occlusal plane.

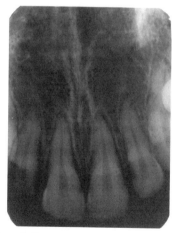

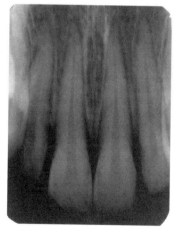

Figure 8–6

Foreshortening of maxillary teeth due to increased positive vertical angulation (overangulation) of cone (PID) in bisecting the angle technique. For mandibular teeth, foreshortening would be due to increased negative vertical angulation in relation to the occlusal plane.

Figure 8–7

Elongation of maxillary teeth due to decreased positive vertical angulation (under-angulation) of cone (PID) in bisecting the angle technique. For mandibular teeth, elongation would be due to decreased negative vertical angulation in relation to the occlusal plane.

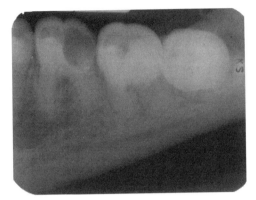

Figure 8–8

Effect of changes in vertical angulation on mandibular teeth.

Figure A

Foreshortening of posterior mandibular teeth due to increased negative vertical angulation. The lower border of the mandible is visible due to foreshortening of the image.

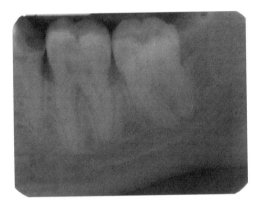

Figure B

Correct length of posterior mandibular teeth. Compare to figure A.

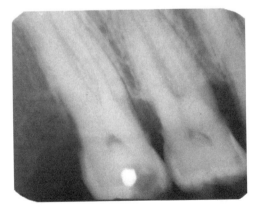

Figure 8–9

Elongation of posterior teeth due to underangulation of x-ray cone in bisecting the angle technique. The apices of teeth are not visible because of the severity of shape distortion.

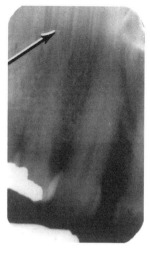

Figure 8–10

Film curving. Shape distortion due to the curving of the film at time of exposure. The superior end of the film was inadvertently curved during patient x radiation. Notice the stretched-out (elongated) bone trabeculae superior to the root apices of the maxillary teeth.

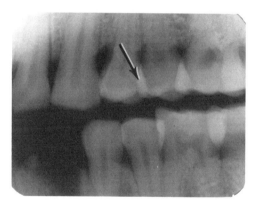

Figure 8–11

Changes in horizontal angulation.

Figure A

Incorrect horizontal angulation results in overlapping of contact points of premolars.

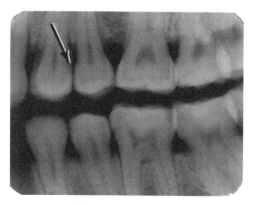

Figure B

Correct horizontal angulation results in visible contact points of premolars.

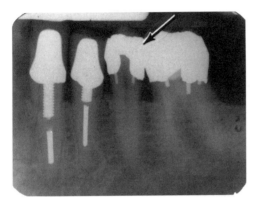

Figure 8–12

Illusion produced by changes in horizontal angulation.

Figure A

Illusion of a closed contact point between the second premolar and first molar due to incorrect horizontal angulation.

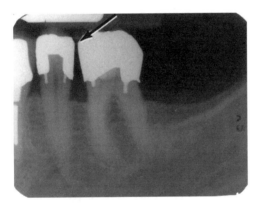

Figure B

Open contact point visible when correct horizontal angulation is used.

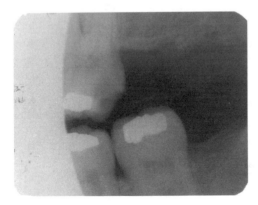

Figure 8–13

Cone-cut caused by improper alignment of circular cone (PID) with film packet. The cone of radiation did not cover the whole area of interest. The clear portion of the film was not exposed to xrays.

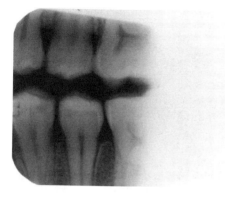

Figure 8–14

Cone-cut caused by improper alignment of rectangular cone (PID) with film packet. The clear portion of the film was not exposed to xrays.

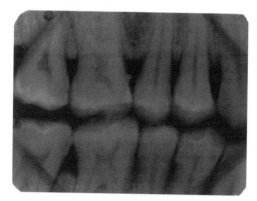

Figure 8–15

Bent film. The black lines caused by creasing the film packet at the four corners produced breaks in the emulsion.

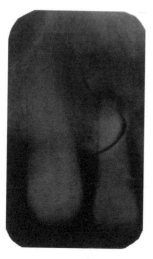

Figure 8–16

Bent film. Film was accidentally crimped when inserting it into the slot of the bite-block. Similar small crescent-shaped images have been erroneously interpreted by many authors as fingernail pressure marks. Clinically, it is difficult to produce fingernail pressure marks on a film.

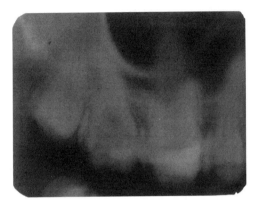

Figure 8–17
Blurred image due to
movement of the film,
patient, or tubehead.

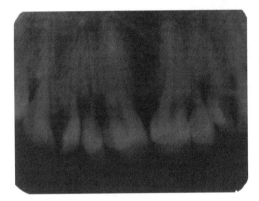

Figure 8–18
Double exposure. The film
was exposed twice,
resulting in a double
image.

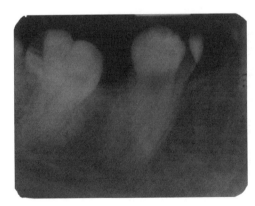

Figure 8–19
Double exposure. The film
was exposed twice,
resulting in a double
image.

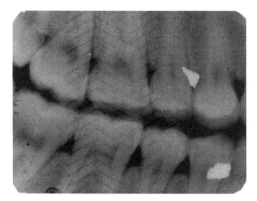

Figure 8–20

Herringbone effect. The film was exposed from the nonexposure surface, that is, the printed back side of film faced the x-ray beam. The film is of low density (light) because the lead film-backing absorbed most of the xrays. Sometimes a honeycomb or tire-track effect may be seen.

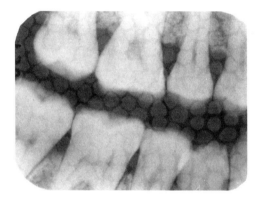

Figure 8–21

Honeycomb effect. Cause is similar to that of the herringbone (or tire- track) effect. The film was exposed from the nonexposure surface. The film is of low density because the lead film-backing absorbed most of the xrays.

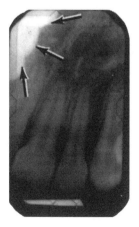

Figure 8–22

The radiopaque images (arrows) are those of the maxillary posterior teeth of contralateral side. During exposure, the upper mesial corner of the film was erroneously placed occlusally to the contralateral maxillary posterior teeth.

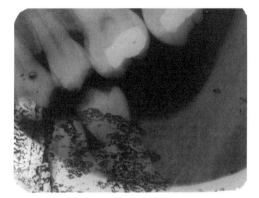

Figure 8–23

Black protective paper stuck to film due to moisture contamination. Failure to blot film moistened with saliva results in the black protective paper (surrounding the film) to stick to the film emulsion. There is also slight cone-cut of the radiograph near the inferior border of the film.

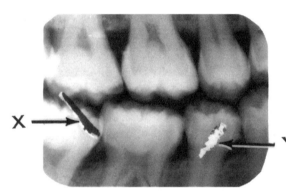

Figure 8–24

The film packet was handled in the darkroom with fingers (gloves) contaminated with saliva. The black mark (X) is the moist black paper stuck to the film. The white clear mark (Y) is the emulsion torn away from the film.

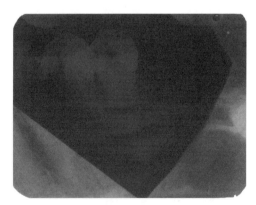

Figure 8–25

Two films stuck together in the automatic processor.

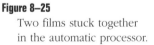

Figure 8–26

A clear film can result from: 1) processing an unexposed film, or 2) placing an exposed or unexposed film first in the fixer (before placing it in the developer), or 3) placing an exposed film in the developer and then leaving it in the fixer for several hours or days.

Figure 8–27

Film exposed to light (or xrays) is completely black after processing.

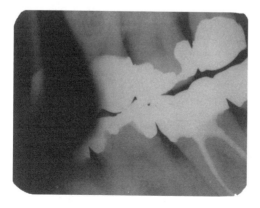

Figure 8–28

Part of the film packet was accidentally opened in daylight and, therefore, became black.

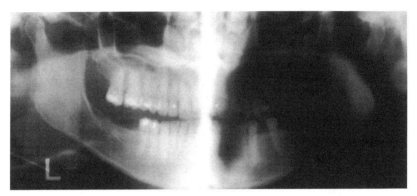

Figure 8-29
Part of the film was exposed to light through a faulty cassette joint and, therefore, turned black.

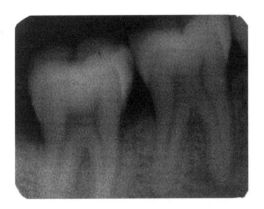

Figure 8–30
Reticulation (orange peel appearance) is caused by sudden extreme temperature changes in manual processing. For example, the developer temperature could be very high and the rinse water temperature could be very cold; the alternate swelling and shrinking of the film emulsion can cause reticulation. This artifact occurs mainly in manual processing; it has not been observed in automatic processing.

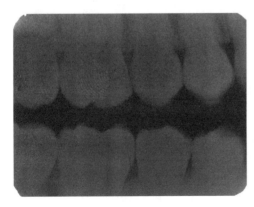

Figure 8–31
Yellow or brown stains on film caused either by insufficient washing of film (fixer remains on film) or by exhausted or contaminated processing solutions. Operator's finger prints are also visible on this radiograph.

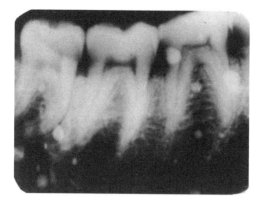

Figure 8–32

Air bubbles clinging on film surfaces during manual processing prevent developer from reducing the emulsion beneath them. These air bubbles cause white spots on the film.

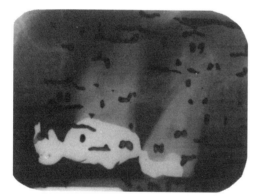

Figure 8–33

Developer artifact. Developer solution splashed on the table top. Unwrapped films were placed on the chemically contaminated table top before being processed in the automatic processor.

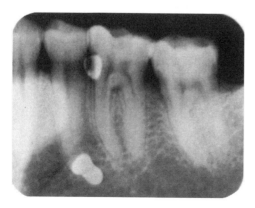

Figure 8–34

Fixer artifact. Fixer solution accidentally splashed on the film before processing. The fixer cleared the undeveloped silver bromide crystals of the film emulsion. (Courtesy Eastman Kodak Company).

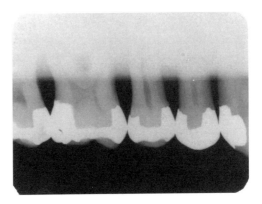

Figure 8–35

In manual processing, the bottom portion of the film was immersed in the developer and then the complete film was immersed in the fixer. This same effect occurs if the level of the developer in the tank is low.

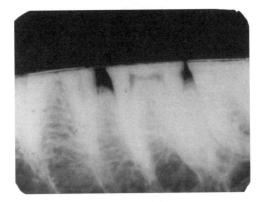

Figure 8–36

In manual processing, if the top portion of the film is green, it means that only the bottom portion of the film was immersed in the developer and in the fixer. If the top portion of the film is black, it means that the whole film was immersed in the developer but only the bottom portion was immersed in the fixer.

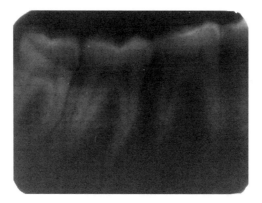

Figure 8–37

Fogged film. The causes of film fog are:

1. Films used beyond the expiration date
2. Films stored at high temperature or high humidity
3. Films inadequately protected from scattered xrays
4. Films processed at excessive time and/or temperature
5. Contaminated or exhausted solutions
6. Darkroom safelight too bright (high bulb wattage)
7. Wrong type of filter in safelight or cracked filter
8. Excessive exposure to safelight
9. Light leaks in darkroom

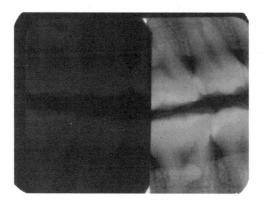

Figure 8–38

Comparison of fogged and unfogged films. (Left) Fogged film; (Right) Unfogged film.

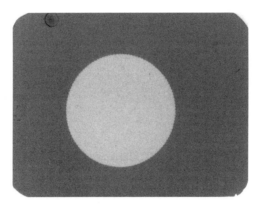

Figure 8–39

Coin test to determine darkroom light safety. In the darkroom, a coin was placed on an unexposed, unwrapped film and left for about two minutes before processing the film. Since the image of the coin is made visible by the surrounding fogged area, the darkroom is not light safe and should be checked for:

1. possible light leaks into the darkroom
2. high wattage of light bulb in safelight
3. wrong filter in safelight
4. too short a distance between safelight and workbench
5. cracked filter in safelight.

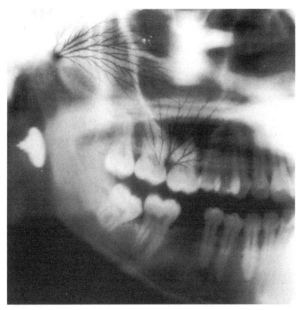

Figure 8–40

Tree-like dark markings produced by a small charge of static electricity as shown on half a panoramic radiograph. Low humidity and dry film are contributing factors. Static electricity is generated by friction from rapid removal of film from its wrapper or from sliding film on the intensifying screen into the cassette.

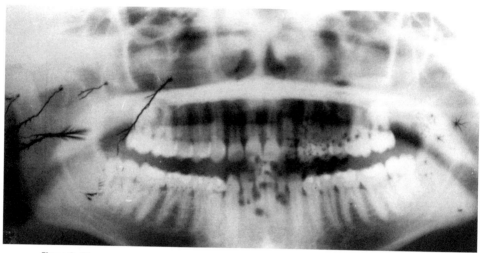

Figure 8–41

Two types of static electricity markings:
1. The smudge or star-like markings (on anterior teeth and left premolars)
2. Tree-like markings (on right ramus)

Although film friction is the most common cause for static electricity markings, sometimes protective latex gloves may be a source of static electricity and produce a black, smudge-like image on a radiograph.

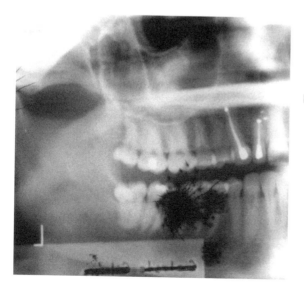

Figure 8–42

Smudge or star-like static electricity markings.

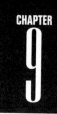

FOREIGN BODIES IN AND ABOUT THE JAWS

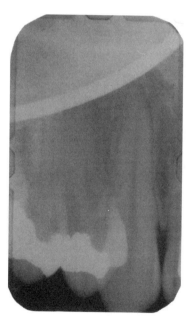

Figure 9–1
Eyeglass lens made of glass (radiopaque) and frame made of metal (radiopaque).

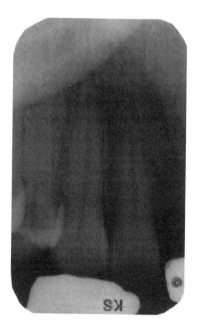

Figure 9–2
Eyeglass lens made of glass (radiopaque) and frame made of plastic (radiolucent).

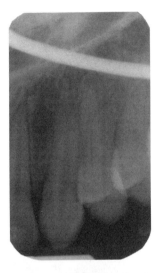

Figure 9–3

Metal frame of eyeglasses (radiopaque). The eyeglass lens is made of plastic (radiolucent).

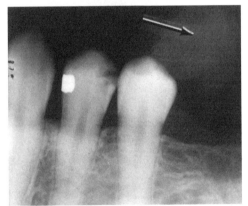

Figure 9–4

Cotton roll. The radiopacity superior to the second premolar is a cotton roll that was used to stabilize the dental instrument. Cotton roll is usually radiolucent but when used in large amounts (thicker), it produces a slightly radiopaque image. It could be misdiagnosed as calcification in the cheek.

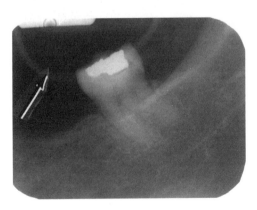

Figure 9–5

Rubber band. The semicircular radiopacity near the crown of the molar is a rubber band that was used around the bite-block and cotton roll to stabilize the dental instrument.

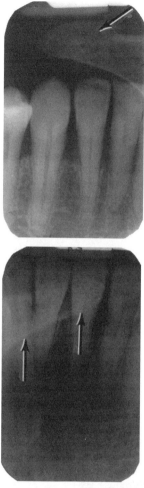

Figure 9–6

Patient's finger accidentally exposed while holding the x-ray instrument rod.

Figure 9–7

Patient's finger accidentally exposed while holding the x-ray instrument rod.

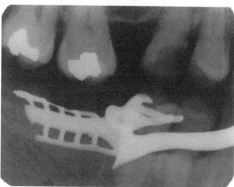

Figure 9–8

Metallic appliance left in patient's mouth during exposure.

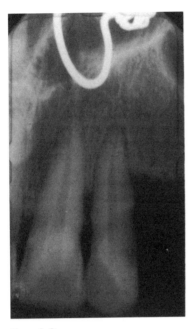
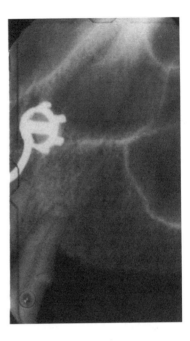

Figure 9–9

Nose ring worn in the ala of the nose. (This custom of wearing a nose-ring is common in some countries.)

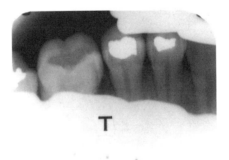

Figure 9–10

Thyroid collar (thyroid shield). The image of the thyroid collar (T) is seen when a patient has a short neck or when a thyroid collar is too large.

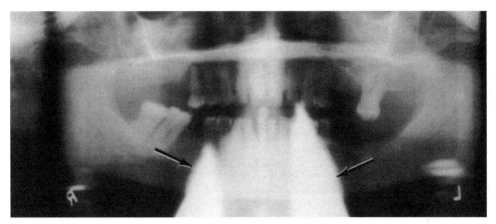

Figure 9–11

Lead apron is visible on a panoramic radiograph when it surrounds the patient's neck. A thyroid shield (collar) will produce a similar image.

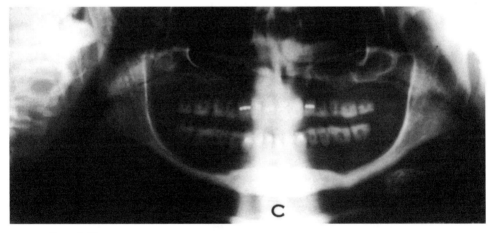

Figure 9–12

Patient's dentures. The patient's maxillary and mandibular dentures were not removed when taking the panoramic radiograph. The cervical spine (C) may be misdiagnosed for a thyroid shield.

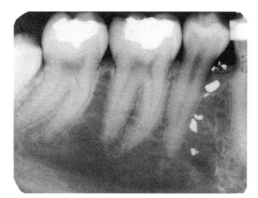

Figure 9–13
Silver amalgam fragments in mucoperiosteum and soft tissue. Clinically, the gray pigmentation of the mucosa is called amalgam tatoo.

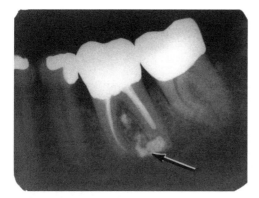

Figure 9–14
Zinc oxide eugenol cement accidentally pushed into the apical region of the first molar during endodontic treatment.

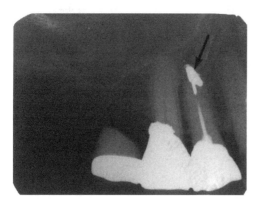

Figure 9–15
Retrograde silver amalgam filling at the apex of the first premolar.

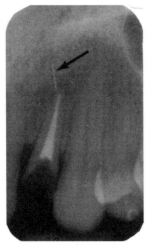

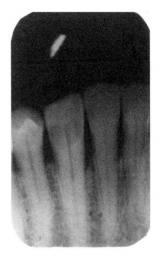

Figure 9–16
Broken endodontic instrument at the periapical region of the maxillary lateral incisor.

Figure 9–17
A metal fragment in patient's lip.

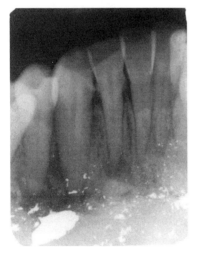

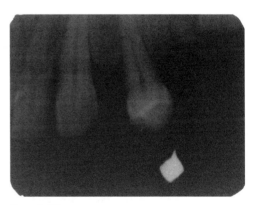

Figure 9–19
Bullet fragment in the soft tissue of the cheek. The root of the maxillary premolar is fractured.

Figure 9–18
Bullet fragments. May be misdiagnosed as amalgam fragments in the mucoperiosteum and soft tissue.

161

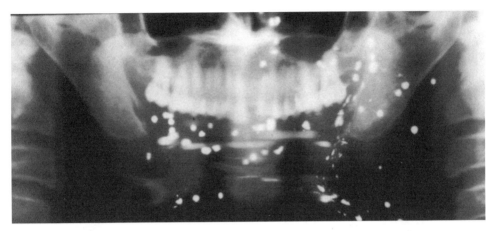

Figure 9–20
Bullet fragments as seen on a panoramic radiograph. The body of the mandible has been surgically excised.

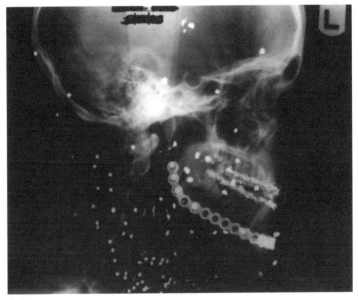

Figure 9–21
Bullet fragments as seen on a lateral skull radiograph. Note the presence of a mandibular reconstruction bone plate.

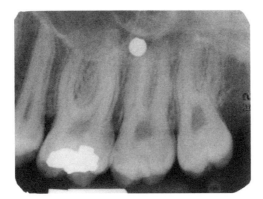

Figure 9–22
Bird shot in the maxilla.

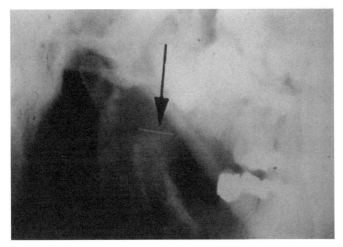

Figure 9–23
Broken hypodermic needle during administration of a mandibular block injection as seen on a lateral jaw radiograph.

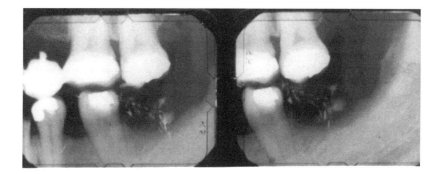

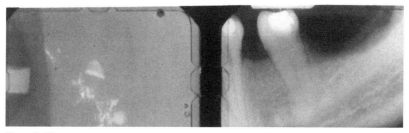

Figure 9–24

Glass fragments in patient's cheek resulting from a car accident eight years earlier. Notice the change in position of the glass fragments with changes in angulation of the x-ray beam.

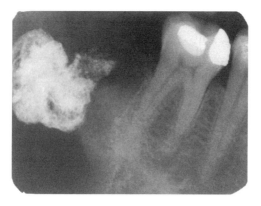

Figure 9–25

Iodoform gauze used as a surgical dressing at the surgically treated site.

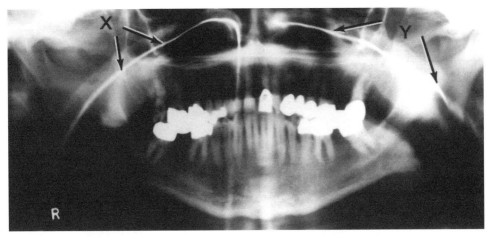

Figure 9–26

Naso-gastric tube (X) inserted into the right nasal passage. The left side shows the ghost image (Y) of the contralateral naso-gastric tube.

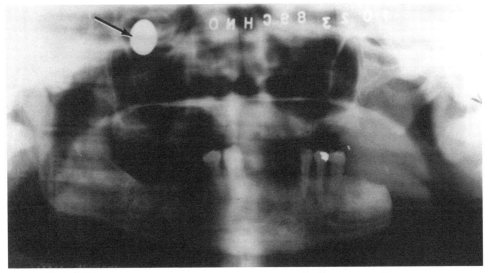

Figure 9–27

Eye implant (right orbit) to which muscles have been attached. The mandibular ramus of the left side was surgically treated because patient had carcinoma of tonsillar fossa.

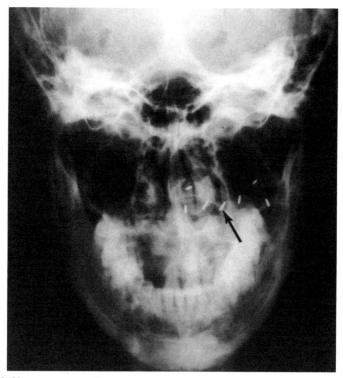

Figure 9–28
Radon seeds implanted for treatment of a tumor.

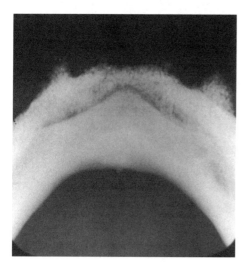

Figure 9–29
Malplacement of hydroxyapatite (hydroxylapatite) for ridge augmentation. The malplaced hydroxyapatite is protruding into the soft tissues.

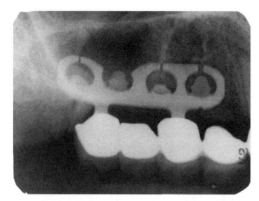

Figure 9–30
Blade implants in maxilla.

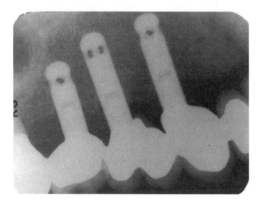

Figure 9–31
Hydroxylapatite coated titanium implants. The implants are used as pier (intermediate) abutments.

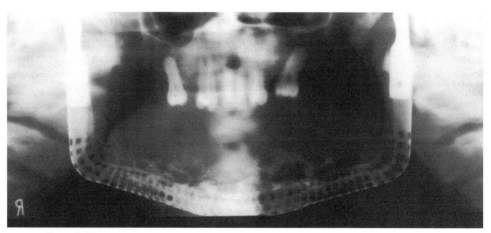

Figure 9–32
Perforated tray for mandibular reconstruction secondary to a tumor.

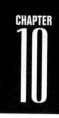

DENTAL ANOMALIES

I. ABNORMALITIES OF DENTAL PULP

Tooth Resorption:

  Physiologic

  Idiopathic

  Pathologic

Pulp Calcifications:

  Pulp Stones

  Secondary/Reparative Dentin

  Pulpal Obliteration

II. ALTERATIONS IN NUMBER OF TEETH

  Anodontia

  Supernumerary teeth

  Mesiodens

III. ALTERATIONS IN SIZE OF TEETH

Macrodontia

Microdontia

IV. ALTERATIONS IN SHAPE OF TEETH

Fusion

Gemination

Concrescence

Dens in dente

Dens evaginatus

Talon cusp

Taurodontism

Dilaceration

Hypercementosis

Enamel pearl

Attrition

Abrasion

Erosion

V. ABNORMALITIES IN POSITION OF TEETH

Submerged teeth

Impacted teeth

Transposed teeth

Ankylosed teeth

VI. Defects of Enamel and/or Dentin

Hypoplasia

Turner's hypoplasia

Amelogenesis imperfecta

Dentinogenesis imperfecta

Dentinal dysplasia

Odontodysplasia

I. Abnormalities of Dental Pulp

TOOTH RESORPTION

Any portion of a tooth may be resorbed as long as such surfaces are associated with other living tissues (for example, bone or pulp). Thus, tooth resorption can occur from the internal surface of a tooth (pulpal surface) or from the external surface of a tooth (enamel or cementum surface). Resorption from the external enamel surface can occur only when the tooth is embedded; that is, surrounded by bone.

From the standpoint of etiology, tooth resorption is classified into three categories:

1. Physiologic root resorption

2. Idiopathic tooth resorption

3. Pathologic tooth resorption

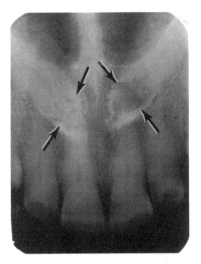

Figure 10–1
Bilaterally impacted canines undergoing resorption of enamel, dentin and cementum (external idiopathic resorption).

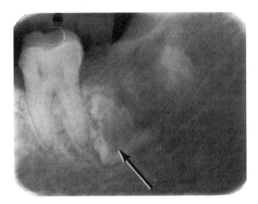

Figure 10–2
Tooth resorption of unerupted third molar (external idiopathic resorption). Ten years ago, this tooth did not show signs of resorption.

PHYSIOLOGIC ROOT RESORPTION

In physiologic root resorption, the roots of a deciduous tooth undergo resorption before the tooth exfoliates. This is a normal physiologic phenomenon. Resorption can occur with or without the presence of a permanent successor tooth. However, if the permanent successor tooth is absent, the resorption of the deciduous tooth is delayed.

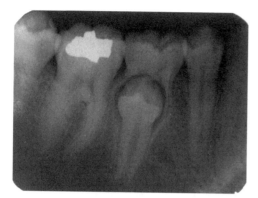

Figure 10–3

Physiologic root resorption of deciduous second molar produced by the succedaneous unerupted second premolar. Root resorption occurs before exfoliation of tooth.

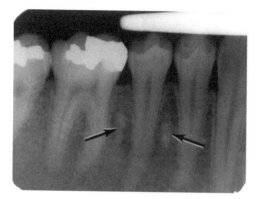

Figure 10–4

Incomplete physiologic root resorption resulting in retained root tips of deciduous second molar.

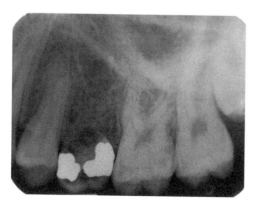

Figure 10–5

Physiologic resorption of deciduous second molar in the absence of the second premolar. Resorption of a deciduous tooth can occur even in the absence of an underlying permanent tooth. However, the resorption may be delayed.

IDIOPATHIC TOOTH RESORPTION

Idiopathic tooth resorption is resorption that occurs either on the internal or external surface of a tooth from an obscure or unknown cause.

(i) Internal (central) idiopathic resorption results in localized increase in the size of the pulp due to idiopathic pulpal hyperplasia. The resorption may continue outwards from the pulpal surface of a crown or a root. This may result in a spontaneous fracture of the tooth. When the internal resorption occurs in a crown, the expanding pulp chamber perforates the dentin and involves the enamel, giving the enamel a pinkish discoloration from the blood vessels being close to the enamel surface. This clinical feature is used to describe it as a pink tooth of Mummery. Internal idiopathic resorption usually involves only one tooth in the dentition.

(ii) External (peripheral) idiopathic resorption can occur on any surface of a crown or root of a tooth. The crown of an erupted tooth cannot undergo external idiopathic resorption because its enamel surface is not surrounded by viable tissue (bone). However, external resorption can occur on the crown of an embedded tooth. If external resorption occurs on the root of a tooth, the resorptive process is followed by a bone filling-in process of the excavated space. If the process of root resorption continues, it may result in the exfoliation of the crown or a spontaneous fracture of the root.

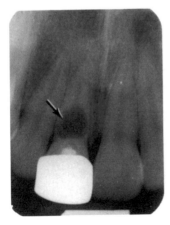

Figure 10–6
Idiopathic internal root resorption of pulp canal of right central incisor. The localized increase in size of the pulp may result in spontaneous root fracture. When a similar resorption occurs in the pulp chamber, the tooth is called a pink tooth because of its clinical appearance.

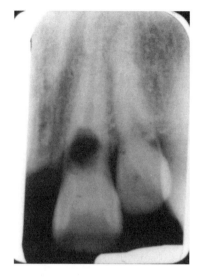

Figure 10–7

Idiopathic internal root resorption of pulp canal of left central incisor. The localized increase in size of the pulp may result in spontaneous root fracture.

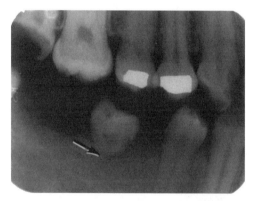

Figure 10–8

Idiopathic external root resorption of the mandibular tooth. If resorption continues, it may result in exfoliation of the crown.

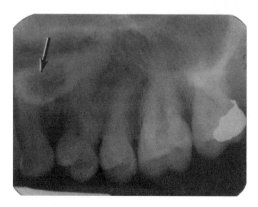

Figure 10–9

Idiopathic external resorption of crown of impacted canine. External idiopathic resorption is usually associated with embedded teeth.

PATHOLOGIC TOOTH RESORPTION

(i) Pressure exerted by an impacted tooth produces a smooth resorbed surface on the adjacent tooth.

(ii) Apical infection produces an irregular resorbed root surface with destruction of the periodontal membrane and lamina dura.

(iii) Neoplasms of expansive nature tend to produce smooth tooth resorption (for example, odontomas and slow-growing ameloblastomas).

Neoplasms of aggressive infiltrating nature tend to produce irregular external tooth resorption.

Neoplasms of extremely aggressive nature have little time for tooth resorption to take place and, therefore, surround the teeth with little or no tooth resorption.

(iv) Trauma produces irregular tooth resorption. However, transient trauma or orthodontic treatment produces a smooth type of resorption. Replanted and transplanted teeth which are not able to reestablish their vascular supply produce an irregular tooth resorption.

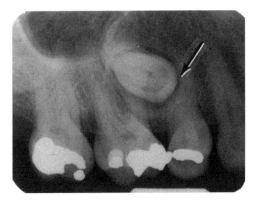

Figure 10–10
Pressure from the impacted second premolar produces a smooth resorbed root surface of the first premolar.

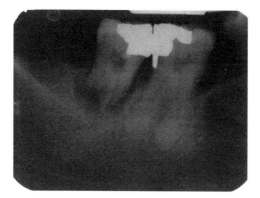

Figure 10–11

Apical tooth infection producing an irregular root surface with destruction of lamina dura and periodontal membrane of the second molar.

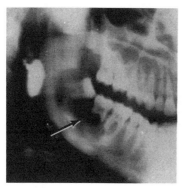 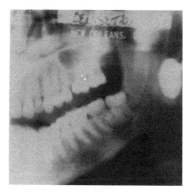

Figure 10–12

The aggressive infiltrating neoplasm in the right mandibular molar region is a fast growing ameloblastoma. It produces a rough external type of root resorption of the second and third mandibular right molars.

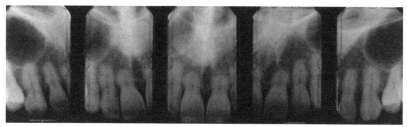

Figure 10–13

Orthodontic treatment produces smooth resorbed roots. All anterior teeth have undergone orthodontic resorption similar to that produced by transient trauma. Teeth have normal vitality with intact periodontal space and lamina dura.

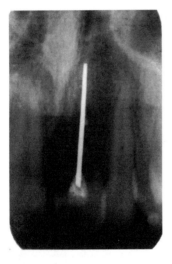

Figure 10–14
The replanted left central incisor tooth has undergone complete root resorption. The silver point of the root canal filling is holding the crown in place. Replantation produces rough and irregular root resorption.

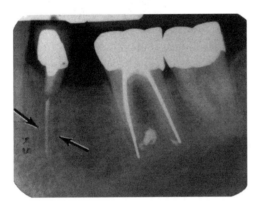

Figure 10–15
The replanted first premolar root has undergone complete resorption. The gutta percha indicates the original location of the root canal.

PULP CALCIFICATIONS

Causes of pulp calcifications are advancing age, dental caries, orthodontic treatment, attrition, abrasion, erosion, dental restorations, trauma, dentinogenesis imperfecta, osteogenesis imperfecta, dentinal dysplasia, and osteopetrosis. Pulp calcification includes pulp stones (denticles), secondary or reparative dentin, and pulpal obliteration (calcific metamorphosis).

Pulp Stones Pulp stones (denticles) radiographically appear as round or ovoid opacities within the pulp. They may be free within the pulp or attached to the inner dental walls. They are not associated with any pain or discomfort. Little or no significance is attached to such stones except that they create a problem during endodontic therapy.

Secondary/Reparative Dentin Secondary or reparative dentin develops as a calcified layer between normal pulp tissue and a large carious lesion. It is frequently associated with the successful use of calcium hydroxide as a pulp-capping material. Some clinicians differentiate between secondary and reparative dentin by using the term secondary dentin to denote deposition of dentin in the pulp chamber as a normal aging phenomenon or as a defense mechanism, and the term reparative dentin to denote deposition of dentin as a result of successful pulp-capping treatment.

Pulpal Obliteration Pulpal obliteration (calcific metamorphosis of dental pulp) is the partial or complete calcification of a pulp chamber and canal. Even though the radiograph may give the illusion of complete obliteration, there is persistence of extremely fine root canal and remnants of the pulp material which make the tooth vital. Teeth that have pulpal obliteration create a difficult endodontic situation when such therapy becomes necessary.

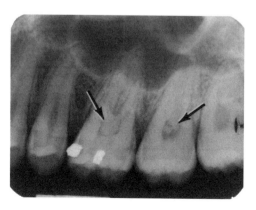

Figure 10–16
Pulp stones (denticles) in the pulp chambers of the first and second molars.

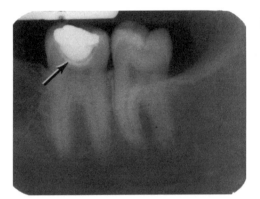

Figure 10–17

Secondary or reparative dentin is present in the restored molar as a result of successful pulp-capping treatment. The secondary dentin (radiopaque) has occurred between the lining of calcium hydroxide (radiolucent) and the pulp chamber.

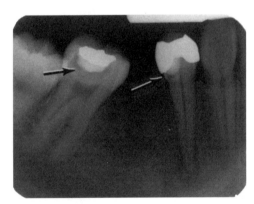

Figure 10–18

Recurrent caries (arrows) under the cement bases of the molar and premolar teeth may sometimes stimulate the formation of secondary (reparative) dentin between it and the pulp chamber.

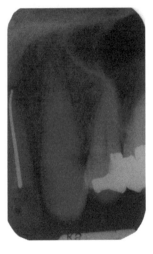

Figure 10–19

Pulpal obliteration (calcific metamorphosis, pulpal calcification) of the canine. The tooth is vital because of the persistence of an extremely fine root canal and remnants of the pulp material.

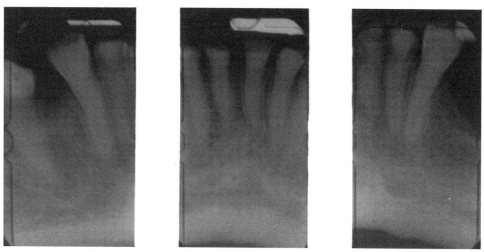

Figure 10–20
Severe attrition may produce generalized pulpal obliteration. The mandibular anterior teeth show calcification of the pulp chambers and root canals as a result of advanced age and attrition.

II. ALTERATIONS IN NUMBER OF TEETH

ANODONTIA

Anodontia denotes congenital absence of all the teeth because of failure of development of tooth germs. Total anodontia is a rare condition but partial anodontia (hypodontia) is more common.

Hypodontia (partial anodontia) denotes congenital absence of one or a few teeth. The affected teeth are usually the third molars and the maxillary lateral incisors. Oligodontia refers to the agenesis of numerous teeth.

Anodontia or hypodontia is often associated with a syndrome known as ectodermal dysplasia.

Pseudoanodontia is the clinical presentation of having no teeth when teeth have either been removed or obscured from view by hyperplastic gingiva.

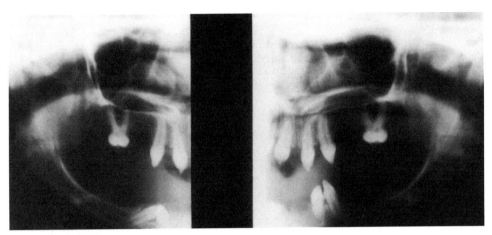

Figure 10–21
Total anodontia of permanent teeth and partial anodontia (hypodontia) of deciduous teeth as a result of agenesis of teeth. The patient suffered from a syndrome called ectodermal dysplasia.

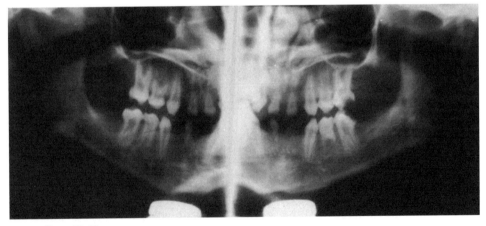

Figure 10–22
Total anodontia of the permanent dentition and hypodontia of the deciduous dentition. This is a rare case in which all the permanent teeth have failed to develop. (Courtesy Dr. P. Schneider).

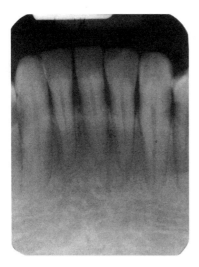

Figure 10–23
Hypodontia. Absence of an incisor tooth. Presence of only three incisors.

SUPERNUMERARY TEETH

Supernumerary teeth (hyperdontia) are additional teeth, over and above the usual number for the dentition. Supernumerary teeth occur as isolated events but are also found in Gardner's syndrome, cleidocranial dysostosis syndrome, and in cases of cleft palate (or cleft lip).

Supernumerary teeth that occur in the molar area are called paramolar teeth; and, more specifically, those that erupt distally to the third molar are called distodens or distomolar teeth. Also, a supernumerary tooth that erupts ectopically either buccally or lingually to the normal arch is sometimes referred to as peridens (plural—peridentes).

The order of frequency of supernumerary teeth is: the mesiodens, maxillary distomolar (fourth molar), maxillary paramolar (buccal to first molar), mandibular premolar, and maxillary lateral incisors.

Some clinicians classify additional teeth according to their morphology: 1) supernumerary teeth and 2) supplemental teeth. Supernumerary teeth are small, malformed extra teeth; for example, mesiodens, distomolar and paramolar. Supplemental teeth are extra teeth of normal morphology; for example, extra premolars and lateral incisors.

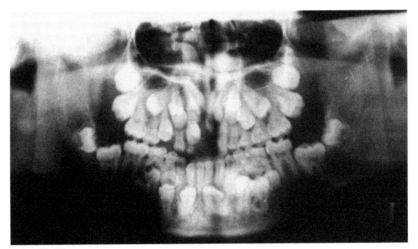

Figure 10–24
Multiple supernumerary teeth in all four quadrants in a developmental disturbance of cleido-cranial dysostosis.

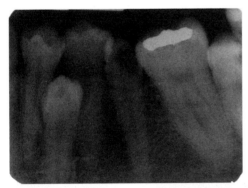

Figure 10–25
Two supernumerary mandibular premolars. One of the two supernumerary premolars is impacted.

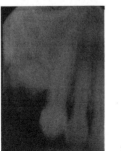
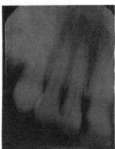
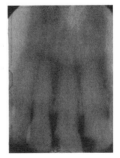

Figure 10–26
Supernumerary lateral incisor. Presence of two lateral incisors in the maxillary right jaw quadrant.

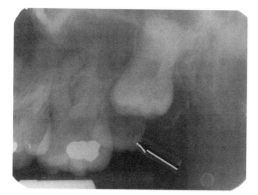

Figure 10–27
Paramolar is a supernumerary tooth in the molar region. The paramolar is obstructing the path of eruption of the third molar.

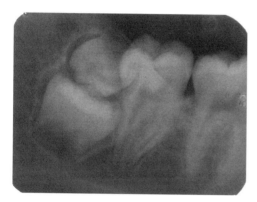

Figure 10–28
The occlusal surface of the paramolar is facing the occlusal surface of the unerupted third molar. May be called, in jest, "kissing molars".

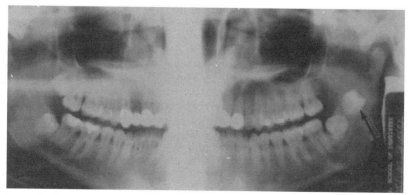

Figure 10–29
Distodens or distomolar is a supernumerary tooth that is distal to the third molar. The distodens is impacted superiorly in the ramus.

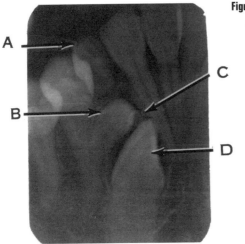

Figure 10–30
A—Deciduous canine
B—Impacted supernumerary tooth
C—Enameloma or odontoma
D—Impacted permanent canine

MESIODENS

Mesiodens (plural-mesiodentes) is a supernumerary tooth that occurs in the anterior maxilla in the midline region near the maxillary central incisors. There may be one or more mesiodentes. The tooth crown may be cone-shaped with a short root or may resemble the adjacent teeth. It may be erupted or impacted, and occasionally inverted. Mesiodens is the most common supernumerary tooth.

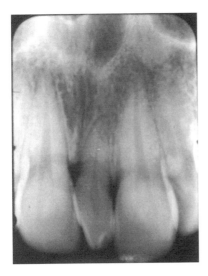

Figure 10–31
An erupted mesiodens between the two maxillary central incisors. The tooth is conical in shape.

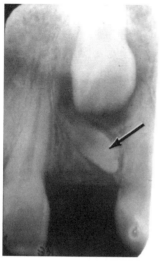

Figure 10–32

An unerupted cone-shaped mesiodens preventing the eruption of the left maxillary central incisor.

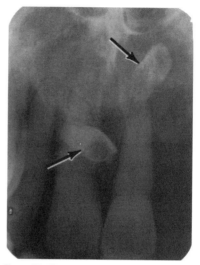

Figure 10–33

Two impacted cone-shaped mesiodentes which exhibit radiolucencies indicating partial resorption. One of the mesiodentes is impacted horizontally and the other is inverted. Mesiodentes occur in the anterior maxilla; they need not be exactly in the midline.

III. Alterations In Size Of Teeth

MACRODONTIA

Macrodontia (megadontia) refers to teeth that are larger than normal. The disorder may affect a single tooth or maybe generalized to all teeth as in pituitary gigantism. In a condition known as hemifacial hypertrophy, teeth on the affected side are abnormally large compared with the unaffected side.

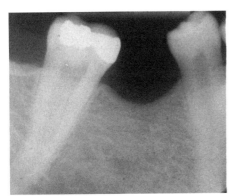 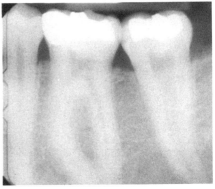

Figure 10–34
Macrodont (megadont) premolars and molars. Macrodontia is a condition in which teeth are larger than normal.

MICRODONTIA

Microdontia refers to teeth that are smaller than normal. Localized microdontia often involves the maxillary lateral incisors or maxillary third molars. The shape of the tooth may be altered as in the case of maxillary lateral incisors which appear as cone-shaped or peg-shaped; hence the term peg laterals. Generalized microdontia may occur in a condition known as pituitary dwarfism.

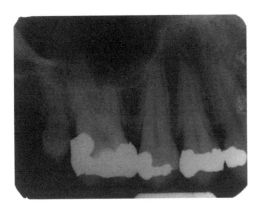

Figure 10–35
Microdontia of maxillary second molar showing reduction in size and in the number of cusps. A microdont is a tooth which is smaller than its normal size.

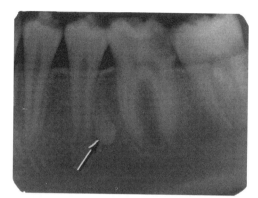

Figure 10–36
Unerupted microdont supernumerary tooth between the roots of the second premolar and first molar.

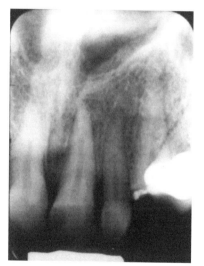

Figure 10–37
Peg lateral incisor. A peg tooth is a form of microdont.

IV. ALTERATIONS IN SHAPE OF TEETH

FUSION (SYNODONTIA)

Fusion is a developmental union of two or more adjacent tooth germs. Although the exact cause is unknown, it could result from contact of two closely positioned tooth germs which fuse to varying degrees before calcification or from a physical force causing contact of adjacent tooth buds. The union between the teeth results in an abnormally large tooth, or union of the crowns, or union of the roots only, and must involve the dentin. The root canals may be separate or fused. Clinically, a fusion results in one less tooth in the dental arch unless the fusion occurred with a supernumerary tooth. The involvement of a supernumerary tooth makes it impossible to differentiate fusion from gemination.

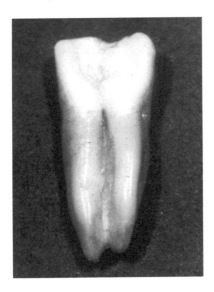

Figure 10–38
    Fusion of the mandibular central incisors. (Courtesy Dr. Eastman collection LSUSD)

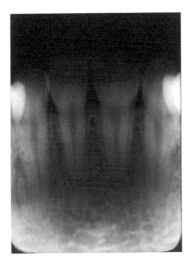

Figure 10–39
    Fusion of mandibular central and lateral incisors on the right and on the left side. The fused teeth are between the right canine and the left canine.

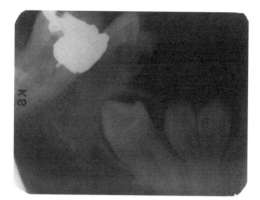

Figure 10–40
Fusion of two unerupted supernumerary teeth. The first premolar is impacted.

GEMINATION

Gemination is the incomplete attempt of a tooth germ to divide into two. The resultant tooth has two crowns, or a large crown partially separated and sharing a single root and root canal. The pulp chamber may be partially divided or may be single and large. The etiology of this condition is unknown. Gemination results in one more tooth in the dental arch. It is not always possible to differentiate between gemination and a case in which there has been fusion between a normal tooth and a supernumerary tooth.

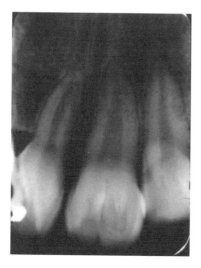

Figure 10–41
Gemination of maxillary left central incisor. The geminated tooth is between the right central incisor and the left lateral incisor.
(Courtesy Dr. J.S. Hubar)

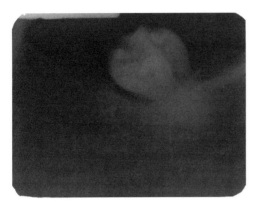

Figure 10–42
Gemination of mandibular molar.

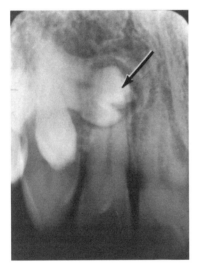

Figure 10–43
Gemination of one of the supernumerary teeth impacted near the apex of the maxillary central incisor.

CONCRESCENCE

Concrescence is a form of fusion occurring after root formation has been completed, resulting in teeth united by their cementum. It is developmental in origin. The involved teeth may erupt partially or may completely fail to erupt. Concrescence is most commonly seen in association with the maxillary second and third molars. It can also occur with a supernumerary tooth. On a radiograph, concrescence may be difficult to distinguish from superimposed images of closely positioned teeth unless additional radiographs are taken with changes in x-ray beam angulation. This condition is of no significance, unless one of the involved teeth requires extraction.

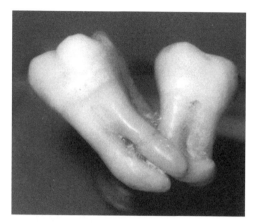

Figure 10–44

Concrescence of mandibular molars. (Courtesy Dr. Eastman collection LSUSD).

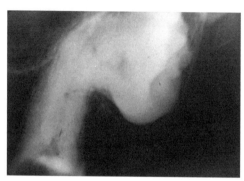

Figure 10–45

Concrescence of maxillary second and third molars. On a radiograph, concrescence is difficult to distinguish from superimposed images of closely positioned teeth unless additional radiographs are taken with changes in x-ray beam angulation.

DENS IN DENTE
(DENS INVAGINATUS, DILATED COMPOSITE ODONTOME)

Dens in dente, also known as dens invaginatus, is produced by an invagination of the calcified layers of a tooth into the body of the tooth. The invagination may be shallow and confined to the crown of the tooth or it may extend all the way to the apex. Therefore, it is sometimes called a tooth within a tooth. In the crown, the invagination often forms an enamel-lined cavity projecting into the pulp. The cavity is usually connected to the outside of the tooth through a very narrow constriction which normally opens at the cingulum area. Consequently, the cavity offers conditions favorable for the development and spread of dental caries. The infection can spread to the pulp and later result in periapical infection. Therefore, these openings should be prophylactically restored as soon as possible after eruption. The maxillary lateral incisor is the most frequently affected tooth. Bilateral and symmetric cases are occasionally seen. Dens in dente can also occur in the root portion of a tooth from the invagination of Hertwig's epithelial root sheath. This anomaly is discovered incidentally on radiographic examination.

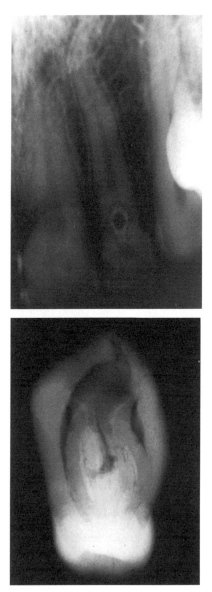

Figure 10–46

Dens in dente (dens invaginatus). The maxillary lateral incisor shows the invagination of the enamel into the tooth pulp chamber. The maxillary lateral incisor is the most frequently affected tooth.

Figure 10–47

Dens in dente shows extensive invagination that involves large portions of the roots and results in open apices.

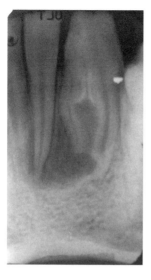

Figure 10–48
> Dens in dente involving crown and root of the mandibular lateral incisor. Observe the apical lesion resulting from infection in the enamel-lined cavity projecting into the pulp.

DENS EVAGINATUS

Dens evaginatus is a developmental condition affecting predominantly premolar teeth. It exclusively occurs in individuals of the Mongolian race (Asians, Eskimos, Native Americans). The anomalous tubercle or cusp is located in the center of the occlusal surface. The tubercle wears off relatively quickly causing early exposure of the accessory pulp horn that extends into the tubercle. This may result in periapical pathology.

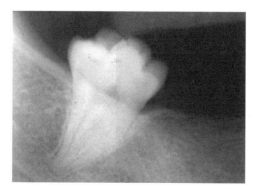

Figure 10–49
> Dens evaginatus exhibiting an anomalous tubercle projecting from the center of the occlusal surface of the molar.

TALON CUSP

The talon cusp is an accessory cusp located on the lingual surface of maxillary or mandibular teeth. Any tooth may be affected but usually it is a maxillary central or lateral incisor. The cusp arises in the cingulum area and may produce occlusal disharmony. In combination with the normal incisal edge, the talon cusp forms a pattern resembling an eagle's talon.

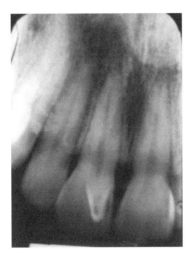

Figure 10–50
Talon cusp arising from the cingulum of the maxillary right central incisor.

TAURODONTISM

Taurodont teeth have crowns of normal size and shape but have large rectangular bodies and pulp chambers which are dramatically increased in their apico-occlusal heights. The apically displaced furcations result in extremely short roots and pulp canals. This developmental anomaly almost always involves a molar tooth. In an individual, single or multiple teeth may be affected either unilaterally or bilaterally. Taurodontism is reported to be prevalent in Eskimos and in Middle Eastern populations. The condition has sometimes been seen in association with amelogenesis imperfecta, tricho-dento-osseous syndrome, and Klinefelter's syndrome. This anomaly is not recognizable clinically, but on a radiograph the rectangular pulp chamber is seen in an elongated tooth body with shortened roots and root canals.

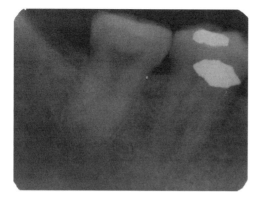

Figure 10–51
Taurodontism involving mandibular second molar which has the characteristic large pulp chamber and short pulp canals.

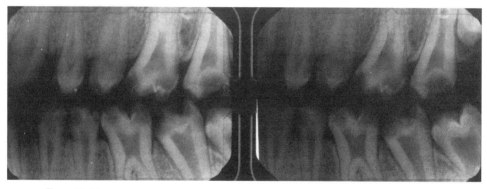

Figure 10–52
A combination of taurodontism and amelogenesis imperfecta. Taurodontism is sometimes seen in association with amelogenesis imperfecta, tricho-dento-osseous syndrome, and Klinefelter's syndrome.

DILACERATION

Dilaceration is an abnormal bend in the root of a tooth. Though the exact cause is not known, it is believed to arise as a result of trauma to a developing tooth which alters the angle between the tooth germ and the portion of the tooth already developed. Dilaceration of roots may produce difficulties during extraction or root canal therapy.

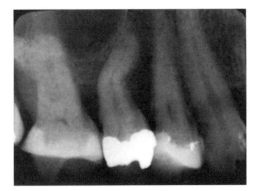

Figure 10–53
Dilacerated root of the
second premolar.
Dilaceration is an
abnormal bend in the root
of a tooth. It is believed to
arise as a result of trauma
to a developing tooth.

HYPERCEMENTOSIS

Hypercementosis is evident on a radiograph as an excessive build-up of cementum around all or part of a root of a tooth. Surrounding this bulbous enlargement of hypercementosis is a continuous periodontal membrane space and a normal lamina dura. In a large majority of instances, hypercementosis affects vital teeth. Generally no cause can be found, but occasionally contributing factors are detected such as periapical inflammation, tooth repair, and teeth that are not in occlusion (impacted, embedded, or without an antagonist). Generalized hypercementosis is sometimes associated with Paget's disease, acromegaly, and pituitary gigantism. No treatment is required.

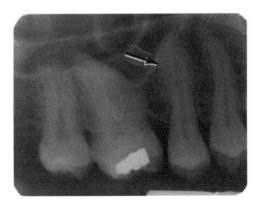

Figure 10–54
Hypercementosis of root of
second premolar.
Hypercementosis is evident
radiographically as an
excessive build-up of
cementum around all or
part of a root of a tooth.

ENAMEL PEARL (ENAMELOMA)

Enamel pearl, also known as enameloma, is an ectopic mass of enamel which can occur anywhere on the roots of teeth but is usually found at the furcation area of roots. The maxillary molars are more frequently affected than the mandibular molars. An enamel pearl does not produce any symptom and when explored with a dental explorer, it may be mistaken for calculus. On a radiograph, the enamel pearl appears as a well-defined round radiopacity.

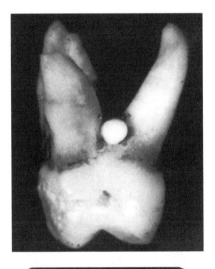

Figure 10–55
Enamel pearl seen at the furcation of the roots of an extracted maxillary molar.

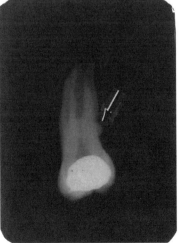

Figure 10–56
Enamel pearl seen on the root surface of a maxillary molar.

199

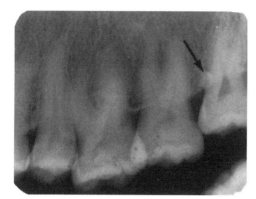

Figure 10–57
Enamel pearl seen at the cemento-enamel junction of the maxillary third molar.

ATTRITION

Attrition is the loss of tooth structure that results from physiologic wear on the incisal and occlusal surfaces of teeth. Chewing habits, bruxism, dental occlusion, and texture of food (tobacco chewing) influence the pattern and extent of attrition. Attrition is an age-related process. Pathologic conditions such as dentinogenesis imperfecta and amelogenesis imperfecta may result in increased attrition. The pulp is usually not exposed because the process of attrition proceeds slowly enough to allow for pulpal recession.

ABRASION

Abrasion is the loss of tooth structure that results from pathologic (mechanical) wear; that is, from friction of a foreign body on a tooth surface. The most common cause of abrasion is vigorous toothbrushing or the use of an abrasive dentifrice. This results in notching of the facial root surfaces adjacent to the gingiva and is most severe on the side opposite to the dominant hand. Abrasion may also occur on the incisal or proximal surfaces from pipe smoking, improper use of toothpicks, misuse of dental floss, biting pencils, cutting thread with teeth, opening bottles or hair pins with teeth, and holding nails with teeth. The pulp is usually not exposed because the process of abrasion proceeds slowly enough to allow for pulpal recession.

EROSION

Erosion is the loss of tooth structure that results from a chemical action not involving a bacterial process. It usually involves all surfaces of teeth but may sometimes involve only one type of surface. In most cases, the teeth are repeatedly in contact with acidic foods and beverages for short or prolonged periods of times to produce surface decalcification which ultimately results in erosion. Many fruit juices and soft drinks have a pH low enough to decalcify enamel; and the habit of sucking lemons, grapefruits or oranges results in continuous exposure to high acidity. Regurgitation of gastric contents as in chronic vomiting, anorexia nervosa, and bulimia syndrome produces generalized lingual erosion of teeth. Many cases of dental erosion are classified as idiopathic in origin because of a lack of definitive proof of chemical action.

Attrition, abrasion, and erosion should be diagnosed by clinical examination, history, and oral habits rather than by the use of radiographs. The radiographic appearance of attrition is that of a smooth wearing of the incisal and occlusal surfaces of teeth whereas that of abrasion depends on the etiology. Toothbrush abrasion appears as well-defined semilunar-shaped cervical radiolucencies. In both cases, the pulps are usually recessed. Erosions are usually not seen on radiographs; however, severe cases appear as radiolucent defects on tooth crowns.

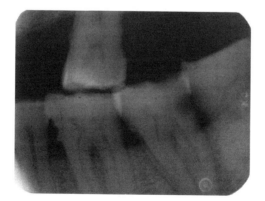

Figure 10–58

Attrition of the posterior teeth with worn out cusps exhibiting flat occlusal surfaces. Attrition is the loss of tooth structure that results from physiologic wear produced on the incisal and occlusal surfaces of opposing teeth coming in contact with one another.

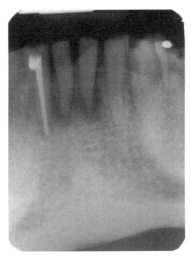

Figure 10–59
Attrition of the mandibular anterior teeth. Pathologic conditions such as dentinogenesis imperfecta and amelogenesis imperfecta may also result in increased attrition.

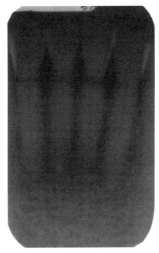

Figure 10–60
Abrasion of the mandibular incisors exhibiting wear at the cervical regions due to vigorous toothbrushing.

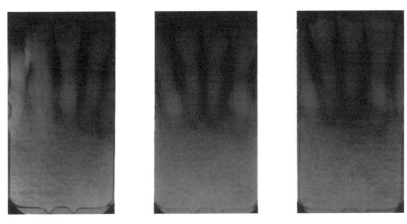

Figure 10–61
Abrasion of the incisal edges of the centrals and laterals. Notice the notchings on the incisal edges. The patient was a seamstress who had a habit of holding pins with her teeth.

V. ABNORMALITIES IN POSITION OF TEETH

SUBMERGED TEETH

A submerged tooth is a retained deciduous tooth (usually a molar) with its occlusal surface at a lower level than the adjoining permanent teeth. In the adjacent areas eruption and alveolar growth continue. The submerged deciduous tooth is usually ankylosed and frequently has a congenitally missing subjacent permanent tooth.

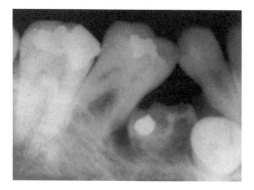

Figure 10–62

Submerged deciduous second molar undergoing resorption of the crown. A submerged tooth is a retained deciduous tooth with its occlusal surface at a lower level than the adjoining permanent teeth. Mesial to the submerged molar is an impacted second premolar in a transverse position.

IMPACTED TEETH

An impacted tooth is a tooth which is prevented from erupting due to crowding of teeth or from some physical barrier or an abnormal eruption path. An embedded tooth is one which has no eruptive force. Any tooth can be impacted; however, it is very rare for the incisors and first molars to be impacted. Mandibular third molar is the most commonly impacted tooth followed by the maxillary third molar, maxillary cuspid and premolar. Tooth impaction may be vertical, horizontal, mesioangular (crown tipped mesially) or distoangular (crown tipped distally). A retained impacted tooth has the potential to develop a dentigerous cyst or a neoplasm (ameloblastoma).

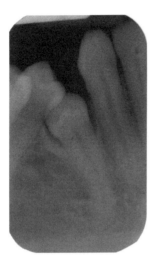

Figure 10–63
Vertical impaction of the first premolar. The crown of the tilted second premolar is preventing the eruption of the first premolar.

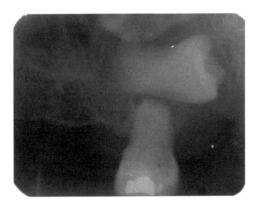

Figure 10–64
Horizontally impacted second molar in the periapical region of the third molar.

TRANSPOSED TEETH

Transposed teeth are two teeth that have exchanged their positions in the dental arch. Abnormal pressures and/or crowding during tooth eruption deflects teeth along an abnormal eruptive path. The permanent canine is most often involved; its position interchanged with the first premolar more often than with the lateral incisor. Second premolars are infrequently found between the first and second molars. Transposition does not occur in primary dentitions.

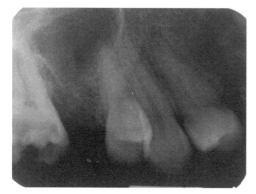

Figure 10–65
Transposition of canine
between the two
premolars. Transposed
teeth are teeth that have
exchanged their positions.

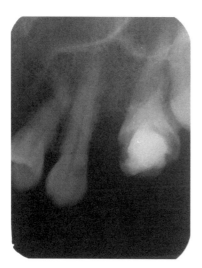

Figure 10–66
Transposed teeth. The canine is
positioned between the premolar
and molar.

ANKYLOSED TEETH

An ankylosed tooth is a tooth in which there is fusion of the cementum
to the surrounding bone. With the loss of the periodontal ligament, bone
and cementum become inextricably mixed, causing union of tooth to
alveolar bone. Ankylosed teeth are extremely difficult to extract and may
sometimes require special skill.

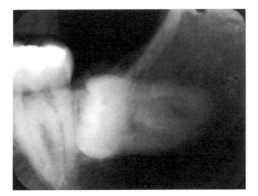

Figure 10–67
Ankylosed third molar. Ankylosis is the union of cementum to the surrounding bone without the intervening periodontal ligament space.

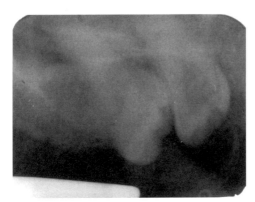

Figure 10–68
Ankylosed maxillary second and third molars. Both the molars are impacted. Also, the roots of the second molar are undergoing resorption.

VI. DEFECT OF ENAMEL AND/OR DENTIN

HYPOPLASIA

Hypoplastic defects alter the shape of teeth. The most commonly observed changes are those resulting in a localized loss of enamel. This loss may take the form of a single pit defect or a series of pits encircling the tooth horizontally. The pits may coalesce to form a groove. The more severe forms of hypoplasia are enamel hypoplasia and enamel hypocalcification. Enamel hypoplasia occurs as a result of a disturbance in the formation of enamel matrix and subsequent deficient amount of enamel tissue. Enamel hypocalcification occurs when a normal amount of enamel matrix is formed but the matrix is not properly calcified.

Causes of hypoplasia:

Local— 1. Trauma (Turner's hypoplasia)

2. Infection (Turner's hypoplasia)

General— 1. Hereditary

a) Dentinogenesis imperfecta

b) Amelogenesis imperfecta

2. Diseases of genetic or idiopathic origin

a) Epidermolysis bullosa dystrophica

b) Cleidocranial dysostosis

c) Osteogenesis imperfecta

3. Prenatal or congenital syphilis

4. Trophic disturbances

a) Gastrointestinal disturbances

b) Infantile tetany

c) Vitamin D, calcium and phosphorus deficiency (rickets)

d) Vitamin C deficiency (infantile scurvy)

e) Exanthematous disease (measles, chicken pox, scarlet fever)

5. Endemic fluorosis

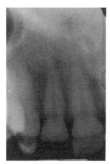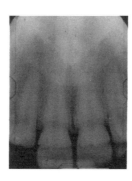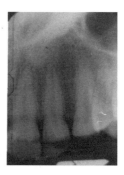

Figure 10–69

Hypoplastic maxillary anterior teeth due to trophic disturbance during the developmental stages. A horizontal groove encircles each tooth.

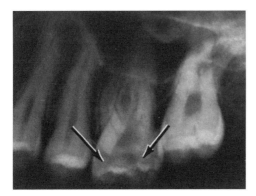

Figure 10–70
Hypoplastic maxillary first molar. The cusps are malformed and have reduced radiodensity of enamel and dentin.

TURNER'S HYPOPLASIA

Turner's hypoplasia, also known as Turner's tooth, is a term used to describe a permanent tooth with a hypoplastic defect to its crown. Localized apical infection or trauma to a deciduous tooth is transmitted to the underlying permanent tooth. If the infection or trauma occurs while the crown of the permanent tooth is forming, the resulting enamel will be hypoplastic and/or hypomineralized. The mandibular bicuspids are most often affected by Turner's hypoplasia since the overlying deciduous molars are relatively more susceptible to infection. Frequently, the maxillary permanent central incisors are affected because of trauma to the overlying deciduous incisors.

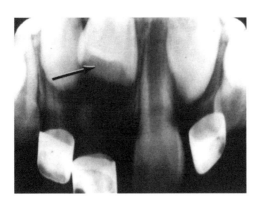

Figure 10–71
Turner's hypoplasia exhibiting hypomineralization of the crown of the unerupted permanent right central incisor. Trauma to the deciduous right central incisor resulted in an inflammatory periapical lesion and thus affected formation of the succedaneous permanent central incisor.

AMELOGENESIS IMPERFECTA

Amelogenesis imperfecta results from a disturbance in the ectodermal layers of developing teeth. It is an hereditary abnormality. There are two types of amelogenesis imperfecta: 1) enamel hypoplasia, in which there is defective formation of enamel matrix, and 2) enamel hypocalcification (hypomineralization), in which the correct amount of enamel is formed but the mineralization of the formed matrix is defective. Amelogenesis imperfecta is hereditary or idiopathic in origin and can affect either the primary or the permanent dentition.

In generalized enamel hypoplasia, the surface of the enamel may be smooth or have pitted hypoplastic areas. The yellowish-brown color of dentin is seen through the thin enamel. The crowns of teeth do not have the usual bulbous contour, resulting in undersized crowns with lack of contact between adjacent teeth. The occlusal surfaces of posterior teeth show occlusal wear caused by abrasion of the thin enamel.

In generalized enamel hypocalcification (hypomineralization), the crowns of teeth are normal in size and shape when they erupt; however, with function, the soft enamel starts to fracture. The hypocalcified enamel and the softer dentin abrade rapidly, resulting in grossly worn down teeth. The increased permeability of the hypomineralized enamel gives it a dark brown color. The enamel has the same radiopacity as the dentin and the two often cannot be differentiated on a radiograph.

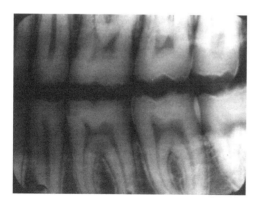

Figure 10–72
Amelogenesis imperfecta, hypoplastic type, shows a thin layer of enamel covering the crowns of the teeth. The occlusal surfaces show wear caused by abrasion of the thin enamel. The proximal surfaces of the crowns do not show the bulbous contour.

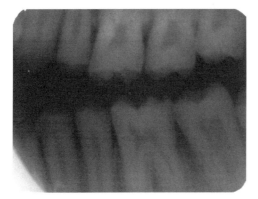

Figure 10–73

Amelogenesis imperfecta, hypoplastic type, reveals absence of enamel. The proximal surfaces of the crowns do not have the usual bulbous contour. The occlusal surfaces show wear caused by abrasion.

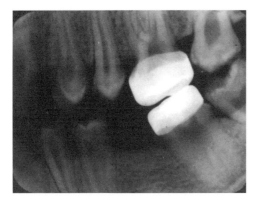

Figure 10–74

Amelogenesis imperfecta, hypoplastic type, reveals tapering undersized crowns with loss of contact between adjoining teeth.

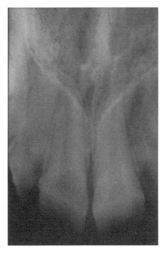

Figure 10–75

Amelogenesis imperfecta, hypocalcified type, shows the crowns with reduced enamel density and rapid abrasion. The enamel has the same radiopacity as dentin.

DENTINOGENESIS IMPERFECTA
(HEREDITARY OPALESCENT DENTIN)

Dentinogenesis imperfecta is a hereditary abnormality in the formation of dentin. The clinical appearance of teeth varies from gray to brownish violet to yellowish brown color, but they exhibit a characteristic unusual translucent or opalescent hue. The crowns fracture easily because of abnormal dentinoenamel junction and the exposed dentin undergoes rapid attrition. Radiographically, the teeth exhibit thin, short roots with constricted cervical portions of the teeth. The pulp chambers and root canals may be partially or completely obliterated. A condition called osteogenesis imperfecta has the same dental characteristics as those of dentinogenesis imperfecta.

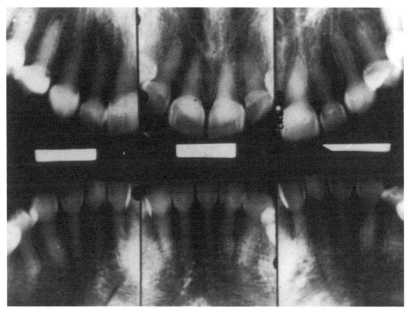

Figure 10–76
Dentinogenesis imperfecta shows thin, short roots constricted in the cervical portions of the teeth. The pulp chambers and root canals are obliterated. Clinically, the teeth had opalescent hue. (Courtesy LSUSD Pediatric Dentistry Department).

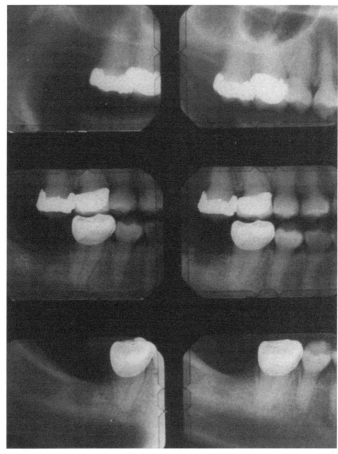

Figure 10–77
Dentinogenesis imperfecta shows obliteration of pulp chambers and root canals of posterior teeth. Clinically the teeth had opalescent hue.

DENTINAL DYSPLASIA

Dentinal dysplasia is a hereditary abnormality. It is subdivided into type I, or radicular type and a more rare type II, or coronal type.

Dentinal dysplasia type I (also known as rootless teeth) affects primarily the root portion of both the deciduous and permanent dentitions. The crowns are of normal color and shape. On a radiograph, the teeth are seen to have very short conical roots with a tendency towards pulpal obliteration. The teeth either exhibit no pulp chambers, or exhibit only residual small crescent-shaped pulp chambers. An abnormality may not be suspected until radiographs reveal pulp and root changes.

Frequently, periapical lesions (chronic abscesses, granulomas, or cysts) occur without any obvious cause; that is, the lesions occur in the absence of caries or trauma to the teeth. Premature tooth loss may occur because of short roots or periapical inflammatory lesions.

Dentinal dysplasia type II (also known as coronal dysplasia) affects primarily the pulp chambers of the deciduous dentition. The crowns of the deciduous teeth are similar in color, shape and contour as those seen in hereditary opalescent dentin (dentinogenesis imperfecta) with premature closure of pulp chambers and canals. The crowns of the permanent teeth are normal but their pulp chambers are often extended and may resemble "thistle-tubes" which frequently contain pulp stones or may be totally obliterated. The roots of teeth with dentinal dysplasia type II are of normal shape and proportion. Periapical radiolucencies are not usually associated with type II, but they are fairly common in type I.

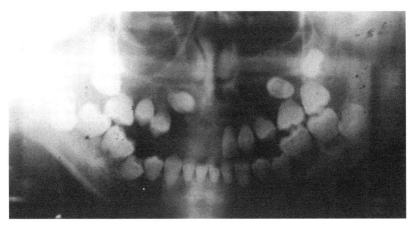

Figure 10–78
Dentinal dysplasia (type I) shows short, poorly developed roots and absence of pulp chambers and root canals.

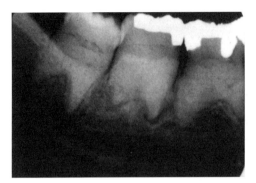

Figure 10–79

Dentinal dysplasia (type I) demonstrates teeth with normal coronal structure, crescents of pulpchambers, short roots, and absence of root canals. Note the presence of numerous periapical lesions.

ODONTODYSPLASIA
(ODONTOGENESIS IMPERFECTA, GHOST TEETH)

Odontodysplasia, or ghost teeth, is a relatively rare developmental abnormality of unknown cause. It results in marked hypoplasia and hypocalcification of enamel and dentin. The cementum is much thinner than normal. The affected teeth are small and have short roots. They are brittle and fracture readily, resulting in pulpal infection. Both dentitions, deciduous and permanent, may be involved. A single tooth or several teeth in a localized area may exhibit the abnormality. The maxillary anterior teeth are affected more than the other teeth. Radiographic appearance shows thin and poorly mineralized enamel and dentin surrounding large pulp chambers and wide root canals. This thinness of enamel, dentin, and cementum gives the teeth the characteristic egg shell appearance and gives rise to the term ghost teeth. Many of these teeth remain unerupted and may, therefore, be mistaken as teeth undergoing resorption.

Figure 10–80

In odontodysplasia, the affected teeth have an eggshell appearance. There is marked hypoplasia and hypocalcification of enamel and dentin. The cementum is much thinner than normal.

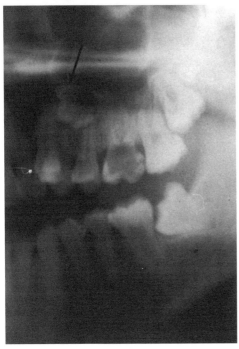

Figure 10–81

Odontodysplasia of a supernumerary tooth at the apices of the maxillary premolars.

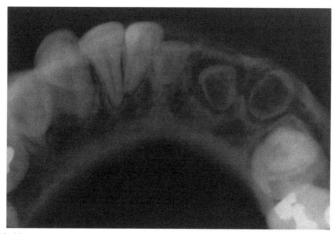

Figure 10–82

Odontodysplasia of the mandibular premolars showing the characteristic eggshell appearance.

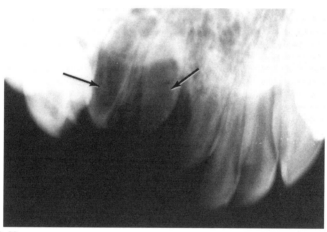

Figure 10–83

Odontodysplasia. The teeth are hypoplastic and hypocalcified. They have the eggshell appearance.

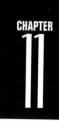

SOFT TISSUE CALCIFICATIONS

Pathologic calcification of soft tissues occurs when calcium and other mineral salts are deposited in a tissue or in a passage. There are three types of pathologic calcifications: 1) dystrophic calcification is that which occurs in degenerating and dead tissues. Calcification of the larval stage of tapeworm (cysticercus) is an example of dystrophic calcification. 2) metastatic calcification is that in which calcium (and other) salts are deposited in previously undamaged tissue as a result of an excess of salts in the circulating blood. Hyperparathyroidism is an example of metastatic calcification which occurs in kidneys and blood vessels. 3) calcinosis is calcification that occurs in or under the skin. Scleroderma, myositis ossificans, and multiple miliary osteomas are examples of calcinosis.

SIALOLITH

A sialolith is a stone (salivary calculus) within a salivary gland or duct. The formation of a sialolith is called sialolithiasis and occurs as a result of precipitation of calcium and phosphate salts around a nidus of mucous or bacterial debris. Sialoliths occur as single or multiple stones and can cause swelling and pain. The pain is experienced during salivary stimulation and is intensified at mealtimes. The accumulation of saliva in the gland produces swelling and the gland becomes enlarged and firm. The pain is produced as a result of the build-up of pressure due to the accumulation of saliva behind the stone. The pain gradually subsides and the swelling diminishes because the stone usually does not completely block the flow of saliva. If a sialolith is small or does not obstruct the flow of saliva, there may be an absence of pain and swelling. More stones are found in the submandibular duct (Wharton's) and gland than in the parotid duct (Stensen's) and gland because of the viscous consistency and mineral content of the saliva from the submandibular gland and the long, irregular length of the Wharton's duct.

The best radiographic projection for visualizing sialoliths in the submandibular duct and gland is the standard mandibular occlusal view. Occasionally, sialoliths are seen incidentally on periapical radiographs, in which case they may be misdiagnosed as osteosclerosis. To differentiate a sialolith from an osteosclerosis, use the Clark's rule of tube-shift technique to localize objects; that is, to find the bucco-lingual relationship. Stones in the parotid duct and gland are best demonstrated by placing a periapical film in the buccal vestibule and x-radiating with a reduced exposure time. Approximately 20% to 40% of all sialoliths are radiolucent. When this is suspected, sialography (injection of a radiopaque dye into the ductal opening and then x-radiating) must be undertaken to visualize the stones. The duct or gland injected with the radiopaque dye shows the radiolucent sialolith as a non-filling defect. A sialolith must be differentiated from other soft tissue calcifications, especially from a calcified lymph node. The latter is usually asymptomatic and sialography may be required to distinguish the two lesions.

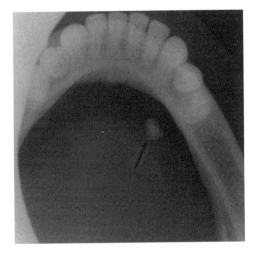

Figure 11–1

Mandibular occlusal projection shows a sialolith (salivary calculus) in the duct of the submandibular gland (Wharton's duct). The patient has a history of pain and swelling in the salivary gland which is intensified at mealtime when saliva flow is stimulated. The pain gradually subsides and swelling diminishes because the stone usually does not completely block the flow of saliva.

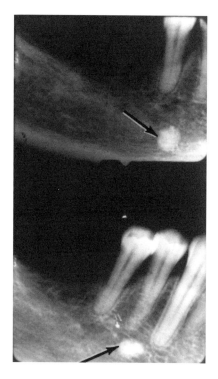

Figure 11–2

On periapical radiographs, the radiopacity may be misdiagnosed as osteosclerosis. To differentiate an osteosclerosis from a sialolith, take two radiographs using different vertical (or horizontal) angulations of the x-ray beam. If the radiopacity changes its position in relation to the adjoining teeth, as shown here, the radiopacity is a sialolith in the floor of the oral cavity (Clark's rule: same lingual, opposite buccal). Another method to identify a submandibular sialolith is to take an occlusal projection.

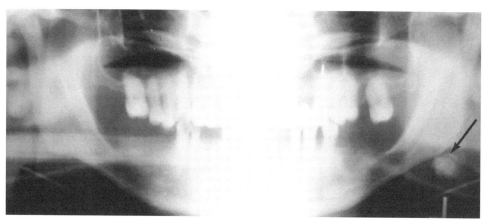

Figure 11–3

A sialolith on a panoramic radiograph may be misdiagnosed as a calcified lymph node. In the absence of clinical signs and symptoms it is difficult to differentiate the two types of calcifications unless a sialogram is made.

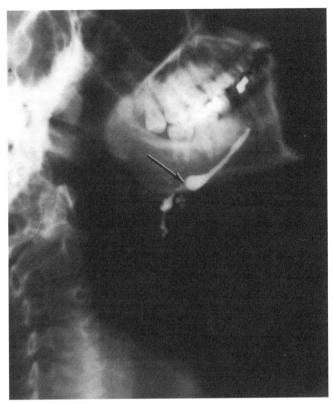

Figure 11–4
Sialogram showing an obstruction in the Wharton's duct preventing the flow of the radiopaque dye into the submandibular salivary gland. The stone (arrow) is blended with the radiopaque dye.

CALCIFIED LYMPH NODE

A calcified lymph node is indicative of a prior chronic infection involving the node. A history of successfully treated tuberculosis is often associated with this calcification. The condition is asymptomatic. It may involve a single node or a chain of submandibular or cervical nodes. The calcified superficial lymph nodes are palpable as bony, hard, round or linear masses with variable mobility. They are often observed on a panoramic radiograph, where they may appear below the inferior border of the mandible and near the angle of the mandible. Calcified lymph nodes are often found incidentally on radiographic examinations. Some may be radiographically projected over the mandibular bone and may be misdiagnosed as osseous lesions.

A calcified submandibular lymph node may be difficult to distinguish from a sialolith. The former is invariably asymptomatic whereas the latter is frequently accompanied by pain and swelling at mealtimes. Sialography may be required to distinguish the two lesions.

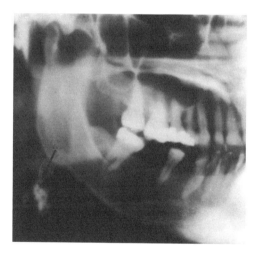

Figure 11–5
Calcified lymph nodes located inferior to the angle of the mandible. Prior chronic infection of the lymph nodes may result in calcification of the nodes. A history of successfully treated tuberculosis is often associated with this calcification. This asymptomatic condition may involve a single node or a chain of nodes.

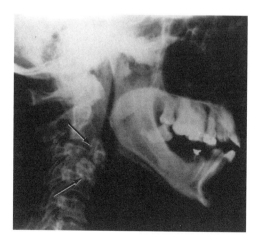

Figure 11–6
A lateral cervical radiograph shows a chain of calcified lymph nodes.

PHLEBOLITH

Phleboliths are calcified thrombi that occur in veins or sinusoidal vessels of hemangiomas involving the soft tissues adjacent to the jaws. On a radiograph they appear as round or oval bodies which may exhibit concentric calcific rings similar to the cross section of an onion. Phleboliths may occur singly or as multiple calcifications. On periapical radiographs, calcifications may be superimposed on the mandible and thus misdiagnosed as osseous lesions within the jaw or as sialoliths.

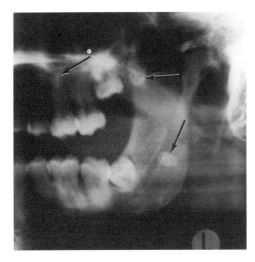

Figure 11–7
Multiple phleboliths superimposed on the mandibular ramus. Phleboliths are calcified thrombi. These calcified masses in blood vessels are associated with hemangiomas found in the cheek.

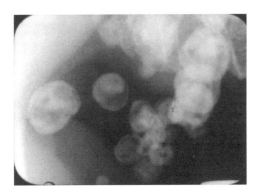

Figure 11–8
Multiple phleboliths of various sizes in cavernous hemangioma of the face. The radiograph is of the patient's cheek.

CALCIFICATION OF ARTERIES

Calcification of the walls of arteries occurs in arteriosclerosis and in secondary inflammatory conditions involving arteries. The calcium salts are deposited within the medial coat of the vessels. Calcification can occur in a number of arteries of the body (iliac, femoral, abdominal aorta, etc.); however, the facial artery is the one often involved in the facial region. Calcified arteries of the cheek and oral cavity may appear as faint images on periapical radiographs. In the Sturge-Weber syndrome (capillary hemangiomas of the face, oral mucosa, and cranium), the cranial hemangiomas often show marked calcification of the blood vessels.

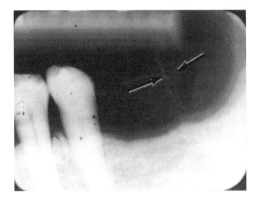

Figure 11–9
　　Calcification of the facial artery. It may occur in arteriosclerosis and represents an inflammatory process.

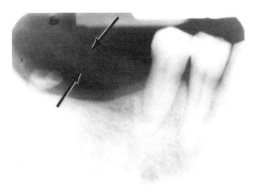

Figure 11–10
　　Calcification of the facial artery. The radiopacity of the artery is the result of deposition of calcium salts within the medial coat of the vessel.

ANTROLITH

A calcified mass in the maxillary sinus is called an antrolith. It is produced by calcification of a nidus which may be a bone chip, root fragment, foreign object, or stagnant mucus in sites of previous inflammation. Most of the antroliths are asymptomatic and are detected incidentally on radiographic examinations. However, on rare occasions when an antrolith continues to grow and become very large, it may be associated with sinusitis. Antroliths must be differentiated from root fragments in the maxillary sinus. A root fragment will show the root anatomy such as the presence of a pulp canal in a cone-shaped (root-shaped) radiopacity. When calcification comparable to an antrolith occurs in the nasal fossa, it is called a rhinolith.

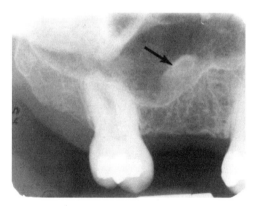

Figure 11–11

Calcified mass in the maxillary sinus is called an antrolith. A foreign object, bone chip, root fragment or stagnant mucus acts as a nidus for calcific deposits. It is usually asymptomatic.

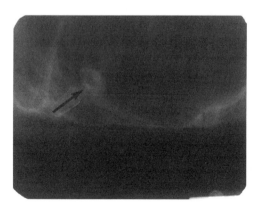

Figure 11–12

Antrolith (stone in maxillary sinus) on the floor of the sinus. It is asymptomatic.

MULTIPLE MILIARY OSTEOMAS OF SKIN (OSTEOMA CUTIS, CALCINOSIS CUTIS)

Multiple miliary osteomas of skin, also known as calcinosis cutis, are situated in the cutis and subcutis. Some of these calcifications are associated with acne or some other form of dermatosis. They are found incidentally on radiographic examinations. They appear as doughnut-shaped radiopacities with radiolucent centers which represent the central marrow cavities. Multiple miliary osteomas are imaged better by placing a dental film in the vestibules and against the inside surface of the cheek and using a reduced exposure time.

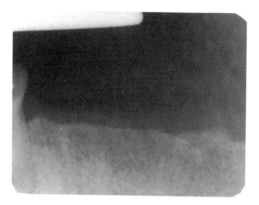

Figure 11–13
Multiple miliary osteomas of skin are soft tissue calcifications of skin. Some are reported to be associated with acne or some other form of dermatosis.

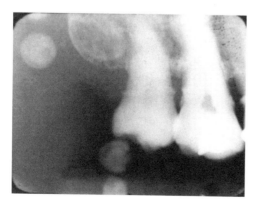

Figure 11–14
Calcinosis cutis showing doughnut-shaped radiopacities.

CALCIFIED STYLOHYOID LIGAMENT AND EAGLE'S SYNDROME

Calcification of the stylohyoid ligament may sometimes be found incidentally on a panoramic radiograph and located posterior to the ramus of the mandible. It may occur unilaterally or bilaterally. In about 50 percent of the cases, the individuals are asymptomatic. In those cases associated with pain and discomfort, the entity is called Eagle's syndrome. The syndrome includes vague pain on mandibular movements such as swallowing (dysphagia), turning the head or opening the mouth, sensation of foreign body in throat, and constant dull ache in the throat. Other symptoms include headache, earache (otalgia), dizziness, pain in temporomandibular joint area and also in the base of the tongue or transient syncope. The symptoms are probably caused by the elongated styloid process impinging on the glossopharyngeal nerve. When the jaws are closed, the pain subsides in some of the cases. It is important for the dentist to be aware that pain associated with calcified stylohyoid ligament may simulate pain associated with that of the temporomandibular joint.

On a radiograph, the calcified stylohyoid ligament appears as a thin, long, tapering radiopaque process extending downwards from the styloid process. Sometimes it may extend up to the lesser horn of the hyoid bone. The farther the mineralized ligament extends towards the hyoid bone, the more likely it is that it will be interrupted by radiolucent joint-like junctions. Surgical resection is required in patients exhibiting symptoms.

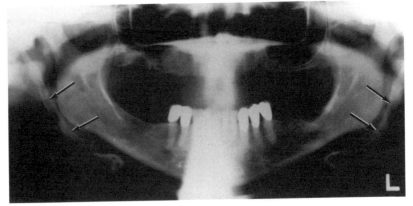

Figure 11–15A

Patient with Eagle's syndrome. The stylohyoid ligaments are bilaterally calcified. Patient complained of constant dull ache in the throat, pain on turning the head, and pain in the vicinity of the temporomandibular joints.

226

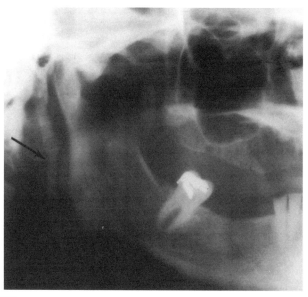

Figure 11–15B

Calcified stylohyoid ligament. Sometimes, this calcification may be associated with Eagle's syndrome. The syndrome produces cervical pain when turning the head, swallowing, and opening the mouth. The patient may have headaches and dizziness.

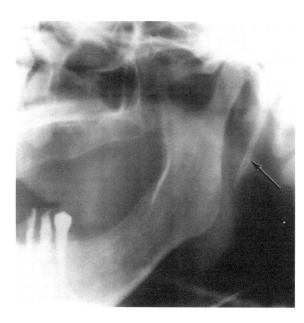

Figure 11–16
Calcified stylohyoid ligament in an asymptomatic patient.

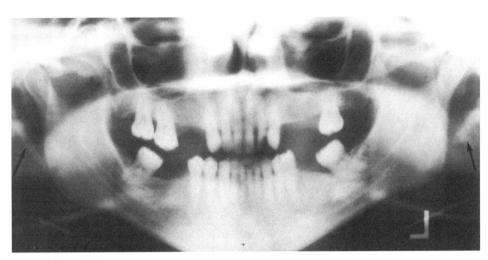

Figure 11–17
Bilateral calcified stylohyoid ligament in a case associated with Eagle's syndrome.

CALCIFIED THYROID CARTILAGE

Calcification of the thyroid cartilage is normal and increases with age. The thyroid and cricoid cartilages have been found to undergo a greater frequency of calcification in the female population, but a higher degree of ossification has been noted in male subjects. (In the hyaline cartilages of the larynx, calcification does not always precede ossification and there is little correlation between the two).

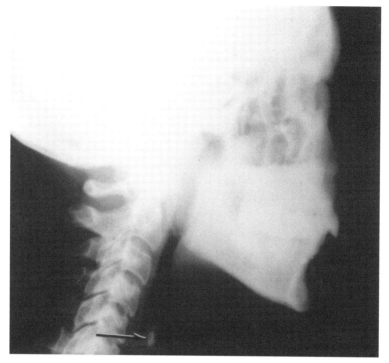
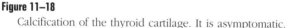

Figure 11–18
Calcification of the thyroid cartilage. It is asymptomatic.

MYOSITIS OSSIFICANS

In myositis ossificans, bony structures such as lamellae, lacunae and marrow are deposited in soft tissue. The cause of this ossification in muscles, ligaments, tendons and fascia is unknown. It may be caused by trauma or heavy muscular strain that occurs in certain occupations and sports. During the healing process, the blood in the traumatized region gets organized and later calcified. The calcification takes place in the connective tissues around the muscles. The digastric, masseter, temporal and sternomastoid are usually involved. The patient finds it difficult to open the jaws when the muscles of mastication are involved. The characteristic radiographic appearance is that of strand-like calcifications along the long axis of the muscle fibers.

CYSTICERCOSIS

Cysticercosis is a helminthic (parasitic worms) disease which completes the larval phase of its life cycle in the pig. When an individual ingests eggs of the (pork) tapeworms from contaminated water or food, the larval form of the tapeworms are hatched in the gastrointestinal tract and enter the vascular and lymphatic systems. They are then deposited in various tissues and organs of the body. At this stage, there is no radiographic evidence of their presence. After their death, the larval spaces are filled with fibrous tissue which later becomes calcified. These calcifications in muscle and subcutaneous tissue are visible on a radiograph as multiple radiopaque ovoid or elliptical objects.

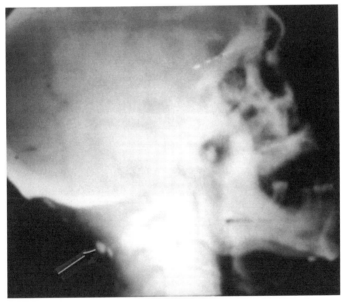

Figure 11–19
Radiograph of patient with cysticercosis. The calcified encysted larvae are seen in the soft tissues at the back of the neck and a single one is seen in the area of Wharton's duct. (Courtesy Dr. E. Cheraskin).

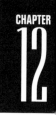

CYSTS OF THE JAWS

ODONTOGENIC CYSTS

Primordial cyst

Dentigerous cyst (follicular)

Radicular cyst (periodontal, dental, periapical, inflammatory, infected)

Lateral periodontal cyst

Residual cyst

Odontogenic keratocyst

Calcifying odontogenic cyst (Gorlin cyst)

NONODONTOGENIC CYSTS

Fissural cysts:

Globulomaxillary cyst

Median mandibular cyst (median alveolar)

Nasopalatine duct cyst (incisive canal cyst, nasopalatine canal cyst)

Median palatal cyst

Nasolabial cyst (nasoalveolar)

Other cysts:

> Traumatic bone cyst (simple bone cyst, hemorrhagic cyst, intraosseous hematoma, idiopathic bone cyst, extravasation bone cyst, solitary bone cyst, solitary bone cavity)
>
> Aneurysmal bone cyst
>
> Mucous retention cyst of maxillary sinus (sinus mucocele, mucoid retention cyst of maxillary sinus, antral retention cyst)
>
> Stafne bone cavity (Stafne bone cyst, lingual cortical defect of the mandible, static bone cavity, latent bone cyst, developmental defect cyst)

A cyst is an epithelium-lined sac containing fluid or semisolid material. In the formation of a cyst, the epithelial cells first proliferate and later undergo degeneration and liquefaction. The liquefied material exerts equal pressure on the walls of the cyst from within. This makes the cyst spherical except when adjoining teeth produce unequal resistance to its growth. Cysts grow by expansion and thus displace the adjacent teeth by pressure. When large, they can produce expansion of the cortical bone. On a radiograph, the radiolucency of a cyst is usually bordered by a radiopaque periphery of dense sclerotic (reactive) bone. The radiolucency may be unilocular or multilocular. Cysts are classified as odontogenic cysts, facial cleft cysts (fissural cysts), and other cysts (nonepitheliated bone cysts, mucous retention cysts and developmental defect cysts).

Odontogenic cysts are those which arise from the epithelium associated with the development of teeth. The source of epithelium is from the enamel organ, the reduced enamel epithelium, the cell rests of Malassez or the remnants of the dental lamina.

Facial cleft or fissural cysts are nonodontogenic cysts that arise from the inclusion of epithelial remnants at the lines of fusion of the various embryonic processes that unite to form the mouth and face. The theory that all the fissural cysts are found at the lines of fissural closure has been found by some authors to be inaccurate. Nevertheless, for convenience these fissural cysts are grouped together in the classification.

Cysts are formed either in bone or in soft tissue. When found in bone, they are called central cysts and when found in soft tissue, they are called peripheral cysts.

PRIMORDIAL CYST

A primordial cyst arises from cystic changes in a developing tooth bud before the formation of enamel and dentin matrix. Since the primordial cyst arises from a tooth bud, the tooth will be missing from the dental arch unless the cyst arose from the tooth bud of a supernumerary tooth. The mandibular third and fourth molar regions are the most common locations for a primordial cyst. It is usually found in children and young adults between 10 and 30 years of age. Radiographically, the primordial cyst is a circular radiolucency with a radiopaque border and found at the site where the tooth failed to develop. Many investigators have reported that most primordial cysts have the same characteristic features as those of odontogenic keratocysts. However, until conclusive proof is established, primordial cysts and odontogenic keratocysts are considered separate entities.

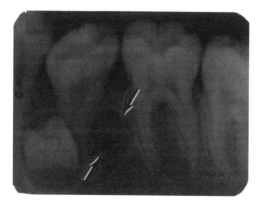

Figure 12–1

Developing tooth follicle of a supernumerary tooth with calcification occurring in the follicle. If calcification had failed to occur, then it would have formed a primordial cyst.

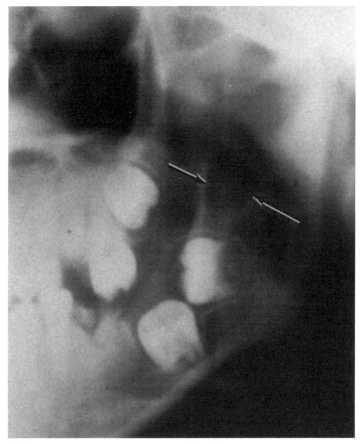

Figure 12–2
Primordial cyst arising from the tooth bud of the fourth molar.

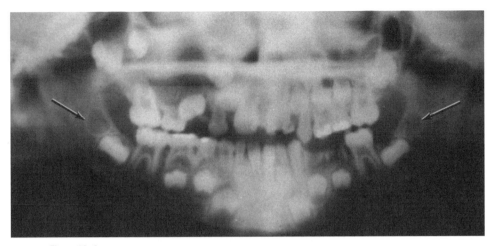

Figure 12–3

Developing tooth follicles of the third molars may be misdiagnosed as primordial cysts.

DENTIGEROUS CYST (FOLLICULAR CYST)

A dentigerous or follicular cyst is formed from the accumulation of fluid between the reduced enamel epithelium and the completely formed tooth crown or in the layers of the reduced enamel epithelium. The crown projects into the cystic space. The tooth remains unerupted because of the overlying cyst. A dentigerous cyst almost exclusively occurs in the permanent dentition, especially in association with impacted mandibular third molars and with impacted maxillary canines. Sometimes the cyst may be situated on only one surface of the crown. Radiographically, the well-defined radiolucency has a radiopaque border and surrounds the crown of an impacted or unerupted tooth. The dentigerous cyst is found in children and adolescents; the highest incidence is in the second and third decades.

Whenever a radiographic diagnosis of a dentigerous cyst is made, the possibility of it being a mural ameloblastoma, a neoplastic transformation of the epithelial lining of a dentigerous cyst, should also be considered. Other pericoronal radiolucencies that radiographically resemble dentigerous cysts are stated below in the differential diagnosis for consideration. It is, therefore, imperative that the clinician send the enucleated specimen for microscopic examination.

The differential diagnosis of a pericoronal radiolucency includes dentigerous cyst, mural ameloblastoma, odontogenic adenomatoid tumor, odontogenic keratocyst, ameloblastic fibroma, ameloblastoma, and calcifying odontogenic cyst.

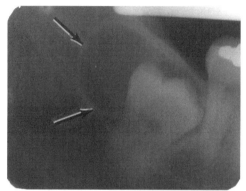

Figure 12–4
Dentigerous cyst (follicular cyst) encircling the crown of the unerupted molar.

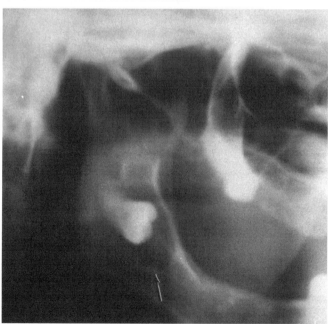

Figure 12–5
Dentigerous cyst encircling the crown of the unerupted mandibular molar.

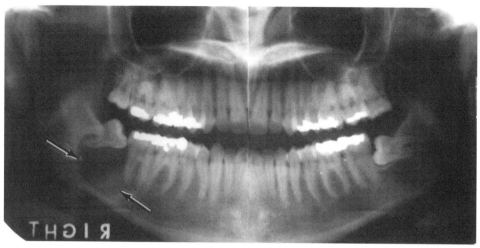

Figure 12–6

Dentigerous cyst attached to the mesial side of the right mandibular third molar.

RADICULAR CYST
(PERIODONTAL CYST, DENTAL CYST, PERIAPICAL CYST, INFLAMMATORY CYST, INFECTED CYST)

The radicular cyst is the most common cyst and is frequently classified as an inflammatory cyst. It has its origin from the cell rests of Malassez which are present in periodontal and periapical ligament, and in periapical granulomas. The main cause of the cyst is infection from the crown of a carious tooth producing an inflammatory reaction at the tooth apex and forming a granuloma. The liquefaction of the apical granuloma produces a radicular cyst. The pulp of the involved tooth is degenerated and the tooth is nonvital. In a multirooted tooth where only one root is associated with the pulpo-periapical pathosis, the tooth will frequently give a vital reaction. Initially, the patient may have had pain from the pulpitis and this is followed by a period without symptoms when the cyst is formed. Therefore, when radicular cysts are found they are usually painless but may sometimes exhibit mild pain or sensitivity to percussion.

Radiographically, the radiolucency is well-circumscribed at the apex of a tooth and usually has a radiopaque border. The lamina dura and periodontal ligament space are destroyed in the region where the lesion is attached to the root. Although a radicular cyst may be misdiagnosed for a granuloma or an abscess, the specific diagnosis is not that critical because all three can be treated by endodontic therapy or with curettage and apicoectomy. (See also Chapter 7, Apical Lesions).

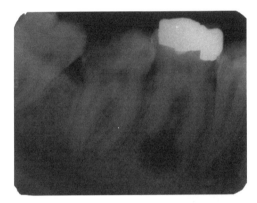

Figure 12–7
   Radicular cyst with a prominent radiopaque border at the apices of the first molar. The first molar is nonvital.

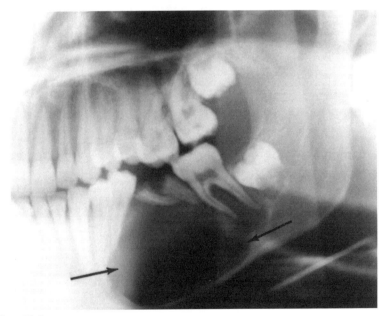

Figure 12–8
   A large radicular cyst at the root apices of the first molar. The lesion has a distinct radiopaque border. An apical inflammatory lesion which is of large size and has well-defined margins is most probably a radicular cyst.

LATERAL PERIODONTAL CYST

The lateral periodontal cyst develops in the periodontal ligament adjacent to the lateral surface of the root of an erupted tooth. It is an uncommon cyst, and when found is often located in the mandibular premolar region, which is an area where supernumerary teeth are frequently found. The lateral periodontal cyst is an asymptomatic cyst. The involved teeth are vital unlike teeth associated with a radicular cyst. On a radiograph, the cyst is seen as a well-defined round or ovoid radiolucency with a radiopaque border. If, on microscopic examination, features of an odontogenic keratocyst are observed then the final diagnosis is that of an odontogenic keratocyst.

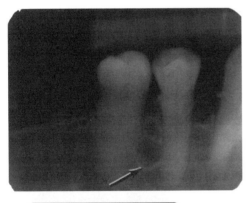

Figure 12–9
Lateral periodontal cyst in its characteristic location in the mandibular premolar region. The teeth are vital.

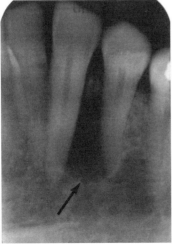

Figure 12–10
Lateral periodontal cyst which histologically had a keratin lining, that is, an odontogenic keratocyst developed from the lateral periodontal cyst.

RESIDUAL CYST

When a tooth having a radicular cyst at its apex is extracted, the radicular cyst is left behind in bone and is now called a residual cyst. A residual cyst can also arise from remnants of the epithelial rests after the extraction of a tooth. This cyst occurs in older individuals; the average age is 50 years. The radiographic appearance is that of a circular radiolucency surrounded by a radiopaque border and occur in an edentulous area. A residual cyst can easily be misdiagnosed as a primordial cyst. The latter arises in lieu of a tooth whereas a residual cyst arises in relation to an extracted tooth.

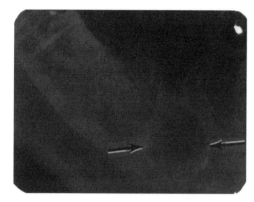

Figure 12–11
Residual cyst at the apex of the socket of the extracted tooth.

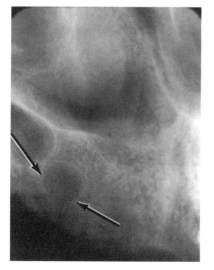

Figure 12–12
Residual cyst in the maxillary canine region. In the differential diagnosis, the possibility of the lesion being a globulomaxillary cyst should also be considered.

240

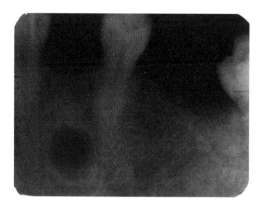

Figure 12–13

Residual cyst at the apical site of the extracted first premolar. In the differential diagnosis, other odontogenic cysts (besides a residual cyst) should be considered, such as: (1) a primordial cyst developed from either the first premolar or a supernumerary tooth, (2) lateral periodontal cyst, (3) odontogenic keratocyst. A radicular cyst should not be considered because the associated second premolar is vital and has an intact periodontal space.

ODONTOGENIC KERATOCYST

An odontogenic keratocyst has a keratinized epithelial lining and an extremely high rate of recurrence. It occurs over a wide range of ages, from 5 to 85 years with the peak incidence being the second and third decades. On a radiograph, a keratocyst may assume the appearance of any odontogenic cyst; for example, primordial, dentigerous, radicular, lateral periodontal or residual cyst. It may produce cortical expansion of bone. The most common site of occurrence is the mandibular third molar and ramus areas. The lesion appears as an unilocular or multilocular radiolucency with a thin radiopaque border of reactive bone. Odontogenic keratocyst shows a striking tendency to recur after enucleation.

An odontogenic keratocyst must be differentiated microscopically and radiographically from other cysts and tumors. If it occurs in the inter-radicular region, it must be differentiated from a primordial cyst, lateral periodontal cyst, calcifying odontogenic cyst and residual cyst. If it occurs pericoronally, it must be differentiated from other pericoronal radiolucencies like dentigerous cyst, mural ameloblastoma, adenomatoid odontogenic tumor, ameloblastic fibroma and calcifying odontogenic cyst. If the odontogenic keratocyst occurs as multilocular radiolucencies it must be differentiated from other multilocular lesions like ameloblastoma, aneurysmal bone cyst, central hemangioma, giant cell lesion of hyperparathyroidism, odontogenic myxoma, central giant cell granuloma, fibrous dysplasia and metastatic tumors of the jaws.

Basal cell nevus syndrome: The occurrence of multiple keratocysts is a characteristic finding in basal cell nevus syndrome. The syndrome, also known as nevoid basal cell carcinoma syndrome, consists of a number of abnormalities including multiple basal cell nevi, multiple jaw cysts, bifid ribs, and intracranial calcifications. The nevoid basal cell carcinomas are usually multiple and involve the face, neck, back, and thorax; often in areas not exposed to the sun. Other anomalies have also been reported: calcification of falx cerebri, mild mandibular prognathism, ocular hypertelorism (eyes widely separated), pits on the palms and soles, characteristic frontal and temporoparietal bossing, and various skeletal anomalies. No single patient has all the listed abnormalities. Basal cell nevus syndrome appears early in life, between the ages of 5 and 30 years.

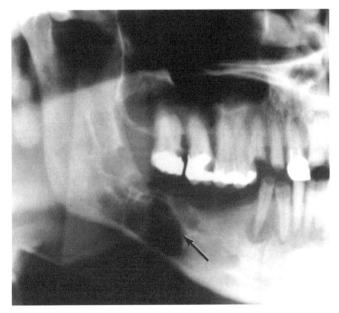

Figure 12–14
An odontogenic keratocyst having a multilocular appearance. It should be differentiated from other multilocular lesions.

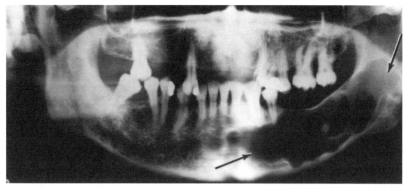

Figure 12–15
An odontogenic keratocyst in the left body and ramus of the mandible and appearing as a large solitary radiolucency.

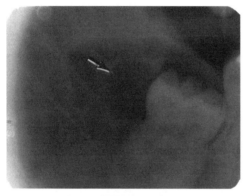

Figure 12–16
An odontogenic keratocyst having a radiographic appearance similar to that of a dentigerous cyst.

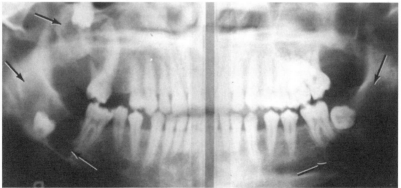

Figure 12–17
Multiple odontogenic keratocysts associated with basal cell nevus syndrome. Basal cell nevus syndrome consists of a number of abnormalities including multiple nevoid basal cell carcinomas, bifid ribs and multiple jaw cysts.

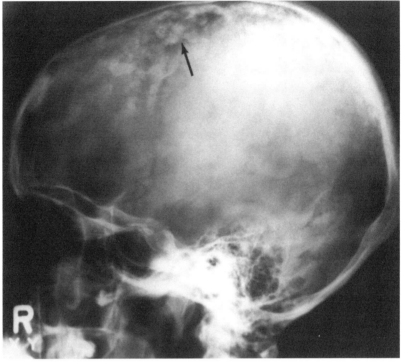

Figure 12–18A
Intracranial calcifications in basal cell nevus syndrome.

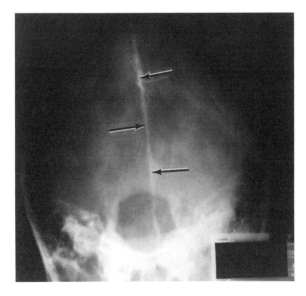

Figure 12–18B
Calcification of falx cerebri in basal cell nevus syndrome. (Courtesy Dr. Jim Weir).

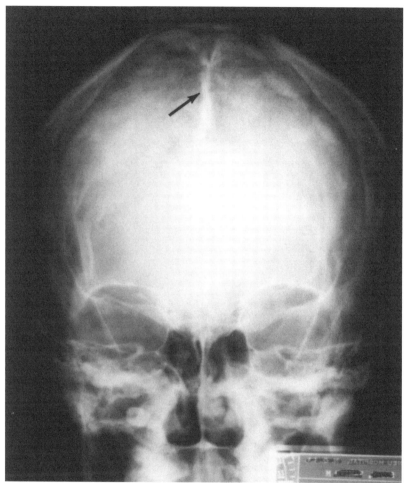

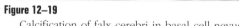

Figure 12–19
Calcification of falx cerebri in basal cell nevus syndrome.

CALCIFYING ODONTOGENIC CYST (GORLIN CYST, KERATINIZING AND CALCIFYING ODONTOGENIC CYST)

Calcifying (epithelial) odontogenic cyst, also called Gorlin cyst, is a rare, slow-growing, benign, tumor-like cyst. It occupies a position between a cyst and an odontogenic tumor since it has some characteristics of a solid neoplasm (continued growth) and some features of a cyst. It should not be confused with the calcifying epithelial odontogenic tumor (Pindborg tumor). This cyst is found in females before the age of 40 years and in males after the age of 40 years. It is equally distributed in the maxilla and the mandible. Most of the calcifying odontogenic cysts are found anterior to the first mandibular molar. On a radiograph, the calcifying odontogenic cyst assumes the appearance of any odontogenic cyst. The radiolucency may be unilocular or multilocular. It is not unusual to find this cyst as a pericoronal radiolucency to an unerupted tooth. Initially, the calcified material may be visible microscopically only, in which case it is completely radiolucent. In other cases, the calcified component may be large enough to occupy the whole lesion. The calcifying odontogenic cyst has been associated clinically with odontomas and ameloblastic fibro-odontomas.

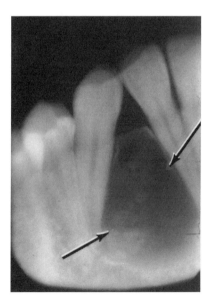

Figure 12–20
Calcifying epithelial odontogenic cyst, also known as Gorlin cyst, showing radiographic evidence of calcified material in the radiolucency.

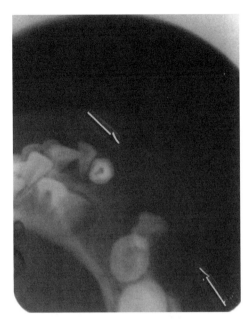

Figure 12–21

Occlusal technique projection of a calcifying epithelial odontogenic cyst showing expansion of the buccal cortical plate. Some of the teeth are displaced by the lesion.

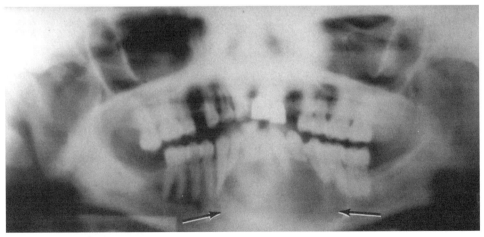

Figure 12–22

Calcifying epithelial odontogenic cyst. This radiolucency does not show any radiographic evidence of calcified material. Microscopically, calcific areas were present in the lesion.

247

GLOBULOMAXILLARY CYST

The globulomaxillary cyst is a fissural cyst originating from epithelial inclusions trapped at the line of fusion between the globular portion of the median nasal process and the maxillary process. This cyst is considered by most pathologists to be not of developmental but of odontogenic origin; that is, it is currently considered to be one of the odontogenic cysts. On a radiograph, the globulomaxillary cyst is seen as an unilocular, inverted pear-shaped (sometimes circular-shaped) radiolucency located between the roots of the maxillary lateral incisor and canine. It causes divergence of the roots of these teeth. The lateral incisor and canine are vital and have intact lamina dura and periodontal ligament space. In edentulous cases, the radiolucent lesion is circular in shape instead of the inverted pear shape.

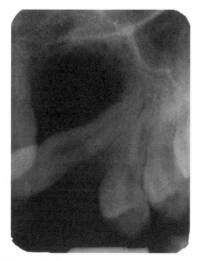

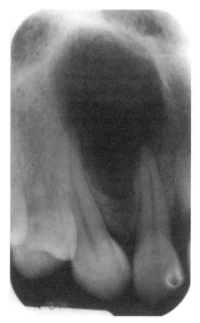

Figure 12–23
Globulomaxillary cyst showing separation of roots of the maxillary lateral incisor and canine. The adjoining teeth (lateral and canine) are vital. Notice the characteristic inverted pear-shaped appearance.

Figure 12–24
Globulomaxillary cyst showing the characteristic inverted pear-shaped appearance. The adjoining teeth are vital.

MEDIAN MANDIBULAR CYST (MEDIAN ALVEOLAR CYST)

Median mandibular cyst is considered to be a very rare cyst. It occurs in the midline of the mandible between the mandibular central incisors from the epithelium trapped in the line of fusion of the paired mandibular processes. Some pathologists believe that it is not of developmental origin but is probably a primordial cyst from a supernumerary tooth, a lateral periodontal cyst, or a radicular cyst. The cyst is asymptomatic and the associated teeth react normally to pulp vitality tests.

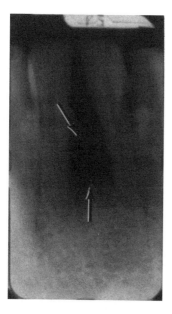

Figure 12–25
Median mandibular cyst is a very rare cyst. The radiolucency (arrows) between the two central incisors is a median mandibular cyst.

Nasopalatine Duct Cyst
(Incisive Canal Cyst, Nasopalatine Canal Cyst)

The nasopalatine duct cyst, also known as incisive canal cyst, is the most common nonodontogenic developmental cyst. It is derived from the embryonic epithelial remnants of the nasopalatine duct which is enclosed within the incisive canal and normally disappears before birth. On a radiograph, the nasopalatine duct cyst is often misdiagnosed as a large incisive foramen. The cyst is located anteriorly in the midline between or above the roots of the maxillary central incisors. The image of the radiopaque anterior nasal spine may in turn be superimposed over the dark cystic cavity, giving it a heart-shaped appearance. Other appearances of the cyst may be round or ovoid. The nasopalatine duct cyst is asymptomatic and usually does not cause any separation or divergence of the roots. The central incisors are vital and have intact periodontal ligament space and lamina dura. Radiopaque stones or concrements are sometimes formed in the incisive canal. The nasopalatine duct cyst rarely becomes large enough to destroy bone; therefore, no surgical treatment is necessary for an asymptomatic small cyst. If the cyst shows signs of infection or shows progressive enlargement, then surgical intervention may be warranted.

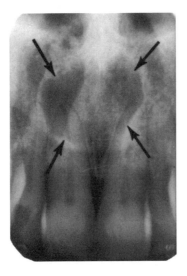

Figure 12–26
Circular-shaped nasopalatine duct cyst (incisive canal cyst) located in the region of the maxillary central incisors. The central incisors are vital and have intact periodontal ligament space and lamina dura.

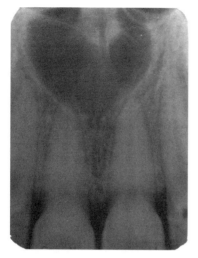

Figure 12–27
Heart-shaped nasopalatine duct cyst. The projection of the anterior nasal spine gives this cyst the characteristic heart-shaped appearance.

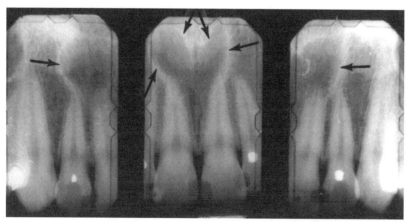

Figure 12–28
Nasopalatine duct cyst having the characteristic heart-shaped appearance.

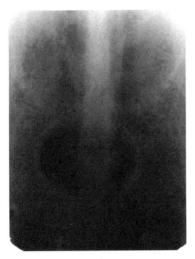

Figure 12–29
Circular-shaped nasopalatine duct cyst in an edentulous patient.

MEDIAN PALATAL CYST

Current views hold that a median palatal cyst is not a separate cyst. A growing trend is to report all maxillary midline developmental cysts as nasopalatine duct cysts, thereby encompassing the so-called median palatal cyst. Many clinicians are of the opinion that the median palatal cyst represents a more posterior presentation of the nasopalatine duct cyst rather than the cystic degeneration of epithelial rests at the line of fusion of the palatine processes of the maxilla.

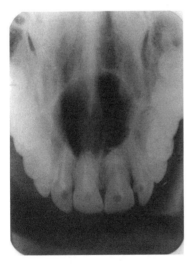

Figure 12–30
Median palatal cyst. Many believe that the median palatal cyst represents a more posterior extension of the nasopalatine duct cyst, and therefore, no distinct lesion such as a median palatal cyst exists.

In this patient, the four incisors were treated endodontically in the mistaken diagnosis that the radiolucency was an inflammatory (pulpo-periapical) lesion.

NASOLABIAL CYST
(NASOALVEOLAR CYST)

Nasolabial cyst, also known as nasoalveolar cyst, is a soft tissue fissural cyst that causes a swelling in the mucolabial fold below the ala of the nose superior to the roots of the maxillary lateral incisor and canine. The cyst may produce elevation of the ala of the nose on that side. The origin of the cyst is from the epithelium entrapped at the fusion of the globular, lateral nasal, and maxillary processes. Nasolabial cyst is not visible on a radiograph because it is a soft tissue cyst. If a radiopaque dye is injected into the cyst, it is clearly visible on a radiograph.

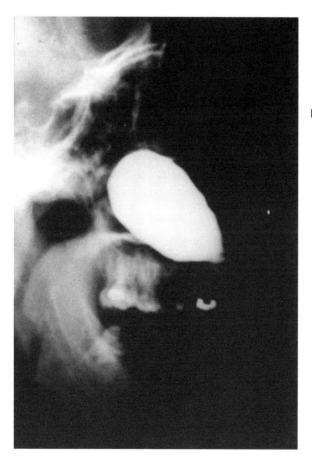

Figure 12–31
Nasolabial (nasoalveolar) cyst is a soft tissue cyst which is made visible on the radiograph by injecting it with a radiopaque dye.

TRAUMATIC BONE CYST
(SIMPLE BONE CYST, HEMORRHAGIC CYST, INTRAOSSEOUS HEMATOMA, IDIOPATHIC BONE CYST, EXTRAVASATION BONE CYST, SOLITARY BONE CYST)

Traumatic bone cyst, also known as simple bone cyst, is not classified as a true cyst because the lesion lacks an epithelial lining. The pathogenesis of this pseudocyst is not known. Many pathologists believe the lesion is a sequela of trauma. Trauma produces hemorrhage within the medullary spaces of bone. In a normal case, the blood clot (hematoma) gets organized to form connective tissue and then new bone. However, if the blood clot for some reason fails to organize, the clot degenerates and forms an empty cavity or a cavity sparsely filled with some serosanguineous fluid and blood clots. It is then called a traumatic bone cyst. Most patients are unable to recall any past history of a traumatic injury to the jaws.

Traumatic bone cyst is a painless lesion having no signs and symptoms and normally does not produce cortical bone expansion. The lesion shows a strong predilection for adolescents and individuals under 40 years of age. The most frequent site of occurrence is the mandibular posterior region and to a lesser extent the mandibular anterior region. Another relatively frequent site is the humerus and other long bones. The involved teeth are vital. The traumatic bone cyst is usually discovered incidentally on radiographic examination. The lesion appears as a well-delineated radiolucency with a radiopaque border. When the radiolucency is adjacent to the roots of teeth, it has a scalloped appearance extending between the roots. The teeth are not displaced and the lamina dura and periodontal ligament space appear intact. If the lesion occurs in areas not associated with the roots of teeth, the well-defined radiolucency may be round or ovoid.

A definitive diagnosis of a traumatic bone cyst can be made only after surgical exploration. However, before surgically entering such a defect, aspiration from the cavity is necessary to rule out the possibility of the lesion being a vascular tumor. After the cyst has been surgically entered, manipulation of the walls of the cavity will induce bleeding into the lesion.

If the cyst is then closed, the blood clot heals and later forms bone. Since the teeth in the involved area are vital, they should not be sacrificed.

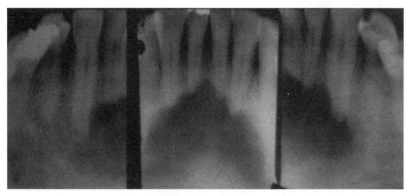

Figure 12–32
Traumatic bone cyst, also known as simple bone cyst, exhibiting the characteristic scalloping between the roots of the mandibular anterior teeth.

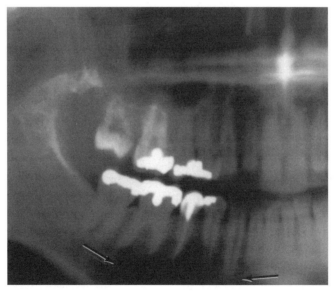

Figure 12–33
Traumatic bone cyst (simple bone cyst) exhibiting the characteristic scalloping in the mandibular premolar and first molar region. The second mandibular premolar was treated endodontically in the mistaken diagnosis that the large radiolucency was an inflammatory apical lesion.

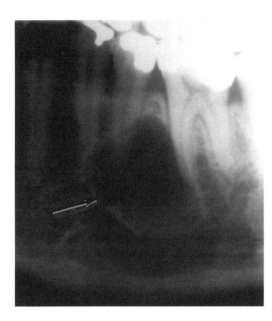

Figure 12–34
Traumatic bone cyst exhibiting a well-defined radiopaque border.

ANEURYSMAL BONE CYST

Aneurysmal bone cyst is not classified as a true bony cyst because the lesion does not have an epithelial lining. It can occur in almost any bone of the skeleton but is more frequent in the spinal column and in the long bones. This abnormality occurs in adolescents and young adults. The cause of this pseudocyst is unknown but some clinicians believe it to be associated with trauma, although most patients fail to give such a history of trauma. Current opinion is that it is an exaggerated localized proliferative response of vascular tissue. It is similar to a central giant cell granuloma and contains giant cells which represent an attempt at repair of a hematoma of bone. The lesion consists of fibrous connective tissue stroma containing many cavernous or sinusoidal blood-filled spaces. The rapid growth of the lesion produces expansion of the cortical plates but does not destroy them. The tender painful swelling produces a marked deformity. The swelling is non-pulsatile and on auscultation, no bruit is heard. If the lesion is an aneurysmal bone cyst, blood can be aspirated with a syringe. The lesion may hemorrhage profusely at the time of surgery but may not create any problem because the blood is not under a great degree of pressure. On a radiograph, the lesion appears as a well-circumscribed unilocular or multilocular cystic lesion causing expansion of cortical plates and resulting in a ballooning or blow-out appearance. The radiolucency is traversed by thin septa, giving it a soap bubble appearance. The teeth are vital and may sometimes be displaced with or without concomitant external root resorption.

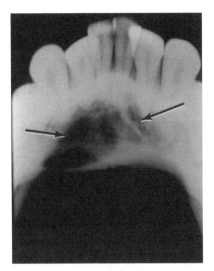

Figure 12–35
Aneurysmal bone cyst in the anterior region of the mandible exhibiting internal septa.

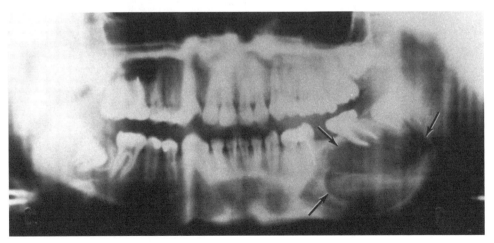

Figure 12–36
Aneurysmal bone cyst producing expansion of the cortical plates.

MUCOUS RETENTION CYST OF MAXILLARY SINUS (SINUS MUCOCELE, MUCOID RETENTION CYST OF MAXILLARY SINUS, ANTRAL RETENTION CYST)

Mucous retention cyst of maxillary sinus is a well-delineated, radiopaque, dome-shaped or hemi-spherical cyst with the antral wall as its base. Most of the mucous retention cysts are located on the floor of the sinus while some are attached to other walls of the maxillary sinus. Although the terms sinus mucous retention cyst and sinus mucocele are sometimes used synonymously, the two lesions are different in etiology and biologic behavior. A sinus retention cyst is a self-limiting nondestructive lesion whereas a sinus mucocele is a destructive lesion which encroaches the adjoining bony structures and landmarks.

The mucous retention cyst represents an accumulation of fluid in the submucosa of the sinus and produces the characteristic radiographic appearance (dome-shaped). Although the cyst arises from soft tissue (sinus mucosa), it is clearly visible on a radiograph because of the radiolucency of the sinus. The lesion may be inflammatory in origin. The fluid appears to be an inflammatory exudate that may on occasion represent extension of adjacent dental infection for which the patient should be evaluated. It has been suggested that allergies and sinusitis probably play a role in their formation since their peak incidence correlates with times of the year when such conditions have a high incidence. Mucous retention cysts are usually asymptomatic but on rare occasions may cause some pain and tenderness in the teeth and face over the sinus. A few of the cysts may persist without change for a long time but a majority disappear spontaneously due to rupture; some may reappear. Those that are of moderate size and asymptomatic can be left untreated. (See also Chapter 17, Maxillary Sinus).

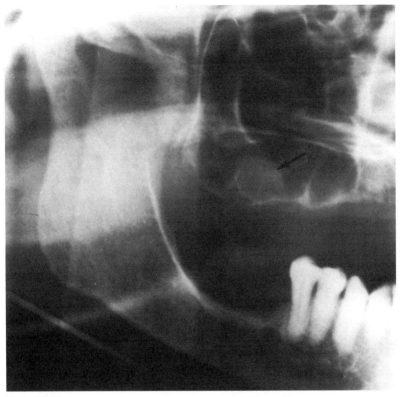

Figure 12–37
Mucous retention cyst seen as a dome-shaped soft tissue radiopacity on the floor of the maxillary sinus.

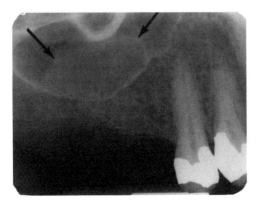

Figure 12–38
Mucous retention cyst on the floor of the maxillary sinus.

STAFNE BONE CAVITY
(STAFNE BONE CYST, LINGUAL CORTICAL DEFECT OF THE MANDIBLE, STATIC BONE CYST, LATENT BONE CYST, DEVELOPMENTAL DEFECT CYST)

Stafne bone cavity, also known as static bone cyst, is a developmental defect of the mandible in the form of a lingual depression in which lies an aberrant lobe of the submandibular salivary gland. The developmental defect is entirely asymptomatic and does not change in size, hence the term static bone cavity. Usually, this defect is unilateral, although on rare occasions bilateral defects have been reported. Stafne bone cavity cannot be palpated manually; it is discovered incidentally during radiographic examination. On a radiograph, the defect is seen in its characteristic location near the angle of the mandible below the mandibular canal.

A similar depression related to the sublingual salivary gland is sometimes found in the anterior region. The Stafne bone cavity appears as a well-defined ovoid or round radiolucency with a wide radiopaque border. To differentiate a Stafne bone cavity from other lesions, sialography of the submandibular gland is performed by injecting a radiopaque dye into the Wharton's duct. If the dye gets carried through the radiolucency, the diagnosis of Stafne bone cavity is confirmed.

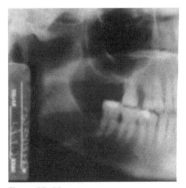 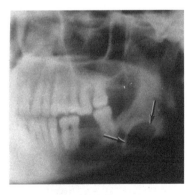

Figure 12–39
Stafne bone cavity is a well-defined cyst-like radiolucency with a radiopaque border. Its characteristic location is near the angle of the mandible, inferior to the mandibular canal.

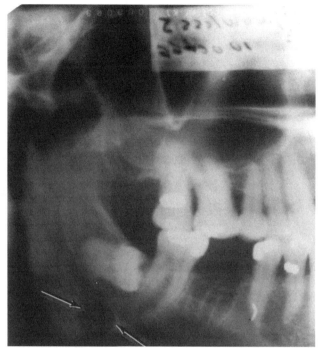

Figure 12–40
Stafne bone cavity near the angle of the mandible, inferior to the mandibular canal.

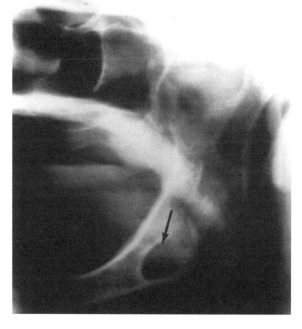

Figure 12–41
Stafne bone cavity located near the angle of the mandible in an edentulous jaw.

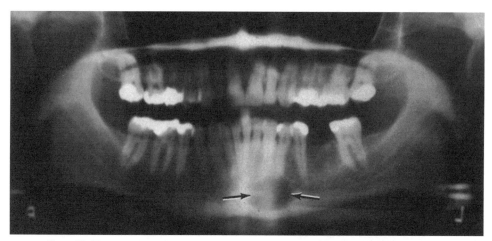

Figure 12–42

Although rare, Stafne bone cavity may be found in the anterior mandibular region. This depression or cavity is related to the sublingual salivary gland.

NORMAL ANATOMY MISDIAGNOSED AS CYSTS

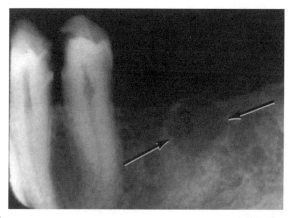

Figure 12–43

Osteoporotic bone marrow defect in the edentulous region. It is an area of hematopoietic or fatty marrow and is seen usually in sites of abnormal healing following extraction, trauma or local inflammation.

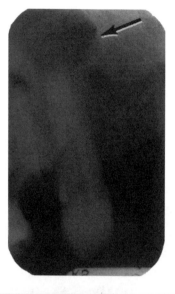

Figure 12–44

Maxillary sinus may be misdiagnosed as a cyst. On a radiograph of the maxillary canine region, the maxillary sinus may be misinterpreted as a radicular cyst. The periodontal ligament space is normal and the tooth is vital.

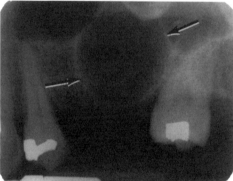

Figure 12–45

Maxillary sinus may be misdiagnosed as a cyst. The crescent shape of the sinus floor and the two septa give the illusion of a cyst.

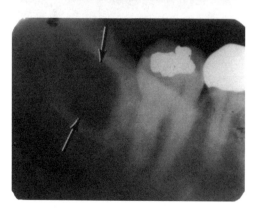

Figure 12–46

Illusion of a cyst. The radiolucency between the radiopaque external and internal oblique lines produces the illusion of a cyst.

DIFFERENTIAL DIAGNOSIS

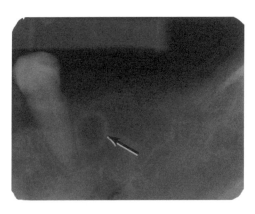

Figure 12–47

Differential diagnosis of an odontogenic cyst in the edentulous site distal to the mandibular premolar: 1) a primordial cyst developed from either a permanent or a supernumerary tooth, 2) residual cyst developed after the extraction of the permanent tooth, 3) lateral periodontal cyst, 4) odontogenic keratocyst. The lesion is not a radicular cyst because the associated premolar is vital and has an intact periodontal space.

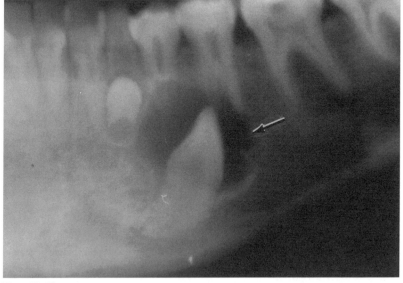

Figure 12–48
Differential diagnosis of a pericoronal radiolucency associated with an anterior tooth. The radiolucency around the crown of the mandibular impacted canine may be: 1) dentigerous cyst, 2) mural ameloblastoma, 3) odontogenic adenomatoid tumor, 4) odontogenic keratocyst, 5) ameloblastic fibroma, 6) calcifying epithelial odontogenic cyst (Gorlin cyst).

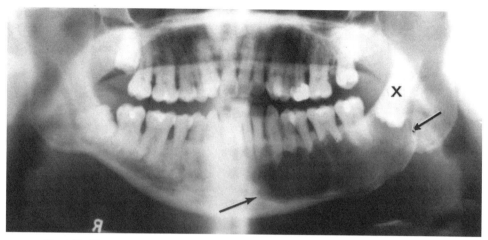

Figure 12–49

Differential diagnosis of a pericoronal radiolucency associated with a posterior tooth. The radiolucency around the crown of the displaced mandibular impacted third molar (X) produces an expansion of the cortical bone. The radiolucency may be: 1) dentigerous cyst, 2) mural ameloblastoma, 3) ameloblastoma, 4) odontogenic keratocyst, 5) ameloblastic fibroma, 6) calcifying epithelial odontogenic tumor (Pindborg tumor).

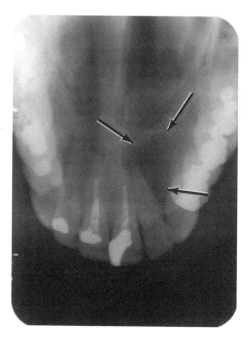

Figure 12-50

Differential diagnosis of a solitary cyst-like radiolucency between the maxillary lateral incisor and canine: 1) globulomaxillary cyst, 2) radicular cyst, 3) odontogenic adenomatoid tumor, 4) odontogenic keratocyst, 5) palatal cleft.

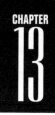

OSTEOMYELITIS

Suppurative osteomyelitis

Garré's osteomyelitis (periostitis ossificans, proliferative osteomyelitis)

Tuberculous osteomyelitis

Syphilitic osteomyelitis

Actinomycotic osteomyelitis

Osteoradionecrosis

SUPPURATIVE OSTEOMYELITIS

Osteomyelitis is an inflammatory reaction of bone to infection which originates from either a tooth, fracture site, soft tissue wound or surgery site. The dental infection may be from a root canal, a periodontal ligament or an extraction site.

Suppurative osteomyelitis can involve all three components of bone: periosteum, cortex, and marrow. Usually there is an underlying predisposing factor like malnutrition, alcoholism, diabetes, leukemia or anemia. Other predisposing factors are those that are characterized by the formation of avascular bone; for example, therapeutically irradiated bone, osteopetrosis, Paget's disease, and florid osseous dysplasia. Osteomyelitis is more commonly observed in the mandible because of its poor blood supply as compared to the maxilla and also because the dense mandibular cortical bone is more prone to damage and, therefore, to infection at the time of tooth extraction.

Acute osteomyelitis is similar to an acute primary abscess in that the onset and course may be so rapid that bone resorption does not occur and, thus, a radiolucency may not be present on a radiograph. Clinical features include pain, pyrexia, painful lymphadenopathy, leukocytosis, and other signs and symptoms of acute infection. Later, after approximately two weeks, as the lesion progresses into the chronic stage, enough bone resorption takes place to show radiographic mottling and blurring of bone. A sclerosed border called an involucrum forms around the affected area. The involucrum prevents blood supply from reaching the affected part. This results in the formation of pieces of sequestra or necrotic bone surrounded by pus. A fistulous tract may develop by the suppuration perforating the cortical bone and periosteum. The fistulous tract discharges pus onto the overlying skin or mucosa.

The radiopacity of the sequestra and the radiolucency of the pus give rise to the characteristic worm-eaten radiographic appearance. Radiographs also aid in locating the original site of infection such as an infected tooth, a fracture, or infected sinus.

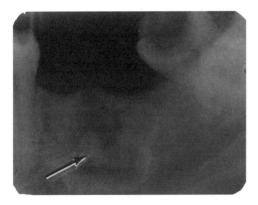

Figure 13–1
Chronic suppurative osteomyelitis of dental origin. The lesion discharged pus into the oral cavity. Note the radiopaque sequestra (arrow) surrounded by the radiolucent suppuration.

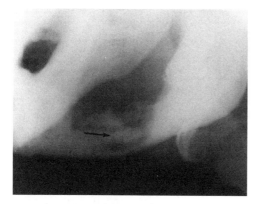

Figure 13–2

Chronic suppurative osteomyelitis demonstrating a worm-eaten appearance of the body of the mandible. Note the radiopaque sequestra surrounded by the radiolucent suppuration and a radiopaque involucrum. The patient had fetid breath.

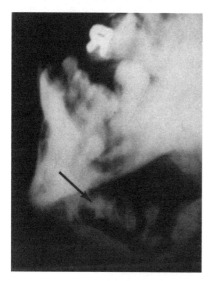

Figure 13–3

Chronic suppurative osteomyelitis of dental origin. The radiopaque sequestrum (arrow) is surrounded by the radiolucent suppuration. (Courtesy Dr. A. Wuehrmann and Dr. L. Manson-Hing).

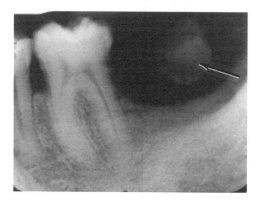

Figure 13–4

Sequestrum that has floated into the soft tissues. Patient gave a history of a problematic tooth extraction several years ago which resulted in clinical complications.

GARRÉ'S OSTEOMYELITIS (PERIOSTITIS OSSIFICANS, OSTEOMYELITIS WITH PROLIFERATIVE PERIOSTITIS)

Garré's osteomyelitis or proliferative periostitis is a type of chronic osteomyelitis which is nonsuppurative. It occurs almost exclusively in children and young adults who present symptoms related to a carious tooth. The process arises secondary to a low-grade chronic infection, usually from the apex of a carious mandibular first molar. The infection spreads towards the surface of the bone, resulting in inflammation of the periosteum and deposition of new bone underneath the periosteum. This peripheral formation of reactive bone results in localized periosteal thickening. The inferior border of the mandible below the carious first molar is the most frequent site for the hard, nontender expansion of cortical bone. On an occlusal view radiograph, the deposition of new bone produces an onion-skin appearance.

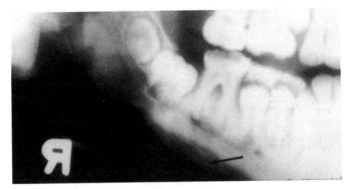

Figure 13–5
Garré's osteomyelitis (proliferative periostitis) demonstrating an expansion of the inferior border of the mandible (onion-skin appearance) caused by the periapical infection of the mandibular first molar.

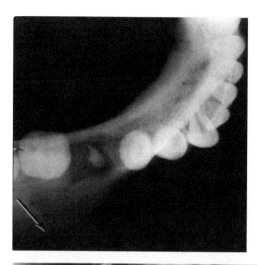

Figure 13–6

An occlusal radiograph of Garré's osteomyelitis showing the buccal expansion of the mandible caused by infection around the root tip of the extracted first molar.

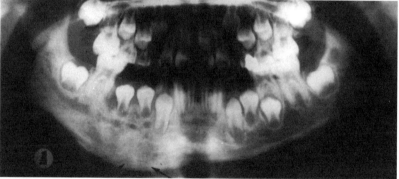

Figure 13–7

Garré's osteomyelitis (periostitis ossificans) exhibiting localized periosteal thickening. The source of infection is not known; it could have been from an exfoliated deciduous molar tooth.

TUBERCULOUS OSTEOMYELITIS

Tuberculosis is a chronic granulomatous disease which may affect any organ, although in man the lung is the major seat of the disease and is the usual portal through which infection reaches other organs. The microorganisms may spread by either the bloodstream or the lymphatics. Oral manifestations of tuberculosis are extremely rare and are usually secondary to primary lesions in other parts of the body. Infection of the socket after tooth extraction can also be the mode of entry into the bone by Mycobacterium tuberculosis. Mandible and maxilla are less commonly affected than long bones and vertebrae. On a radiograph, the appearance of bony lesions is similar to that of chronic suppurative osteomyelitis (worm-eaten appearance) with fistulae formation through which small sequestra are exuded. Periostitis ossificans (proliferative periostitis) can also occur and change the contour of bone. Calcification of lymph nodes is a characteristic sign of tuberculosis.

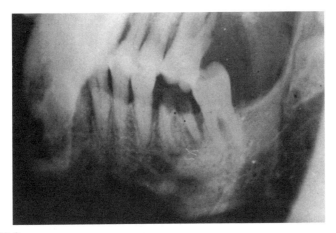

Figure 13–8

Tuberculous osteomyelitis showing the worm-eaten appearance similar to that of a chronic suppurative osteomyelitis (Courtesy Dr. A. Wuehrmann and Dr. L. Manson-Hing).

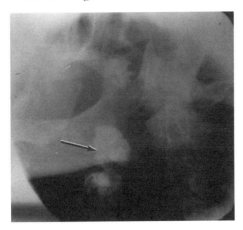

Figure 13–9

Calcified tuberculous lymph nodes (Courtesy Dr. L. Manson-Hing).

272

Syphilitic Osteomyelitis

Syphilis is a chronic granulomatous disease which is caused by the spirochete Treponema pallidum. It is a contagious venereal disease which leads to many structural and cutaneous lesions. Acquired syphilis is transmitted by direct contact whereas congenital syphilis is transmitted in utero. In congenital syphilis, the teeth are hypoplastic; that is, the maxillary incisors have screwdriver-shaped crowns with notched incisal edges (Hutchinson's teeth) and the molars have irregular mass of globules instead of well-formed cusps (mulberry molars). Also, a depressed nasal bridge or saddleback nose occurs because of gummatous destruction of the nasal bones.

Acquired syphilis, if untreated, has three distinct stages. The primary stage develops after a couple of weeks of exposure and consists of chancres on the lips, tongue, palate, oral mucosa, penis, vagina, cervix or anus. These chancres are contagious on direct contact with them. The secondary stage begins 5 to 10 weeks after the occurrence of chancres and consists of diffuse eruptions on skin and mucous membrane. This rash may be accompanied by swollen lymph nodes throughout the body, a sore throat, weight loss, malaise, headache and loss of hair. The secondary stage can also damage the eyes, liver, kidneys and other organs. The tertiary-stage lesions may not appear for several years to decades after the onset of the disease. In this stage of syphilis, the bone, skin, mucous membrane, and liver show gummatous destruction which is a soft, gummy tumor that resembles granulation tissue. Paralysis and dementia can also occur. In the oral cavity, the hard palate is frequently involved resulting in its perforation. The gummatous destruction is painless. Syphilitic osteomyelitis of the jaws is difficult to distinguish from chronic suppurative osteomyelitis since their radiographic appearances are similar.

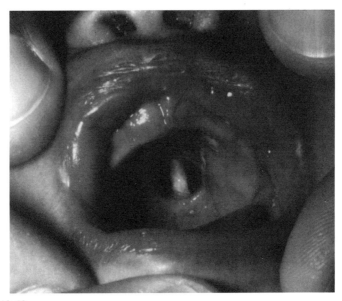

Figure13–10
Syphilitic osteomyelitis of the palate. The gummatous destruction has produced a palatal perforation.

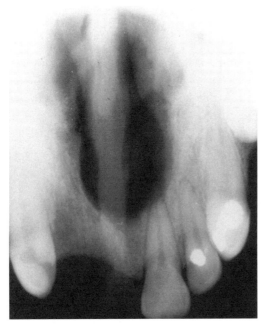

Figure13–11
Radiograph of syphilitic osteomyelitis of the palate. The perforation which is the site of gumma of the hard palate produces a radiolucency which may be mistaken for a median palatine cyst.

ACTINOMYCOTIC OSTEOMYELITIS

Like tuberculosis and syphilis, actinomycosis is a chronic granulomatous disease. It can occur anywhere in the body, but two-thirds of all cases occur in the cervicofacial region. The disease is caused by bacteria-like fungus called Actinomyces israelii. These microorganisms occur as normal flora of the oral cavity, and appear to become pathogenic only after entrance through previously seated defects. The portal of entry for the microorganisms is through the socket of an extracted tooth, a traumatized mucous membrane, a periodontal pocket, the pulp of a carious tooth or a fracture. In cervicofacial actinomycosis, the patient exhibits swelling, pain, fever and trismus. The lesion may remain localized in the soft tissues or invade the jaw bones. If the lesion progresses slowly, little suppuration takes place; however, if it breaks down, abscesses are formed that discharge pus containing yellow granules (nicknamed sulfur granules) through multiple sinuses.

There is no characteristic radiographic appearance. In some cases the lesion resembles a periapical radiolucent lesion. The more aggressive lesion resembles chronic suppurative osteomyelitis. In chronic suppurative osteomyelitis there is usually a single sinus through which pus exudes; however, in actinomycotic osteomyelitis there are many sinuses through which pus and sulfur granules exude.

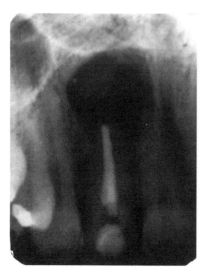

Figure13–12
Actinomycotic lesion similar to radicular cyst. This is not a typical appearance. (Courtesy Dr. J. Weir).

OSTEORADIONECROSIS
(AND EFFECTS OF IRRADIATION ON DEVELOPING TEETH)

In therapeutic radiation for carcinomas of the head and neck, the jaws are subjected to high exposure doses of ionizing radiation (average of 5000 R). This results in decreased vascularity of bone and makes them susceptible to infection and traumatic injury. Infection may occur in irradiated bone from poor oral hygiene, extraction wound, periodontitis, denture sores, pulpal infection or dental treatment. It is, therefore, advisable that a patient scheduled to undergo therapeutic radiation be given dental treatment prior to radiation therapy and that after radiation therapy the patient be taught to maintain good oral hygiene. When infection occurs in irradiated bone, it results in a condition called osteoradionecrosis which is similar to chronic suppurative osteomyelitis. The mandible is affected more commonly than the more vascular maxilla. Therapeutic radiation may affect the salivary glands, producing decreased salivation. The resulting temporary or permanent xerostomia is responsible for radiation caries of teeth and erythema of the mucosa.

A radiograph of osteoradionecrosis shows radiopaque sequestra and surrounding radiolucent purulency similar to that of chronic suppurative osteomyelitis. The two cannot be differentiated radiographically except by the history of therapeutic radiation.

Effects of irradiation on developing teeth depends on the stage of development when irradiation occurs and on the dosage administered. The injured tooth germs may either fail to form teeth (anodontia), exhibit dwarf-teeth, produce agenesis of roots, shortening and tapering of roots, or develop into hypoplastic teeth. The eruption of teeth may be retarded and their sequencing may be disturbed. Other radiation-induced effects may include maxillary and/or mandibular hypoplasia.

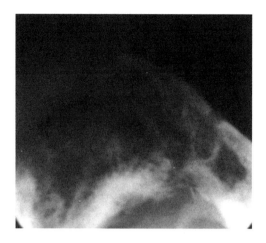

Figure13–13
Occlusal projection of anterior region of mandible showing osteoradionecrosis. Notice the destruction of the trabecular pattern of bone.

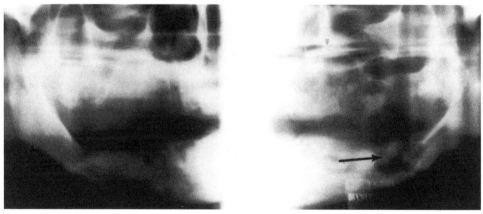

Figure13–14
Osteoradionecrosis of left mandible showing the radiopaque sequestra.

277

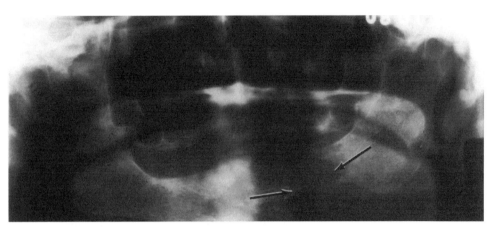

Figure13–15
Osteoradionecrosis of left mandible has resulted in a pathologic fracture.

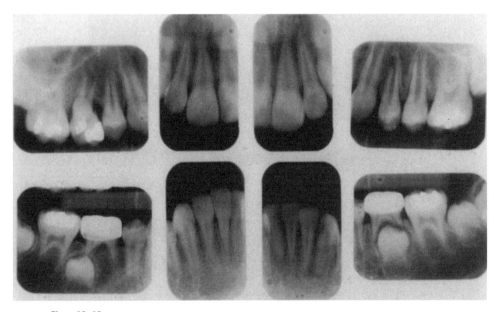

Figure13–16
Dwarfing of teeth as a consequence of radiation therapy (Courtesy Dr. L. Guerra).

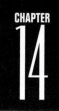

ODONTOGENIC BENIGN TUMORS OF THE JAWS

I. Epithelial Odontogenic Tumors
(With no inductive change in connective tissue)

    1. Ameloblastoma

    2. Odontogenic adenomatoid tumor (Adenomatoid odontogenic tumor)

    3. Calcifying epithelial odontogenic tumor (Pindborg tumor)

II. Mixed Odontogenic Tumors—Epithelial and Mesenchymal
(With inductive change in connective tissue)

    1. Ameloblastic fibroma

    2. Ameloblastic odontoma

    3. Ameloblastic fibro-odontoma

    4. Odontomas

III. Mesenchymal Odontogenic Tumors

    1. Odontogenic myxoma (myxofibroma)

    2. Odontogenic fibroma

    3. Cementifying (ossifying) fibroma

    4. Cementoblastoma

AMELOBLASTOMA

Ameloblastoma is the most prevalent of all the odontogenic tumors combined, the only exception being the odontomas. It is a locally aggressive, slow-growing, epithelial odontogenic neoplasm which arises from remnants of the dental lamina, enamel organ, and cell rests of Malassez. It can also occur from the epithelial lining of a dentigerous cyst, in which case it is called a mural ameloblastoma. The lesion occurs in patients between the ages of 30 to 60 years, predominantly in the fourth and fifth decades. The most favored sites are the mandibular molar region, angle of mandible, and ascending ramus. The tumor is painless and remains asymptomatic as it enlarges. The patient notices a gradual jaw expansion producing facial asymmetry. The cortex is often thinned but is seldom penetrated by the growth. The recurrence rate is high after surgical treatment.

The most common radiographic image is that of multilocular cyst-like radiolucencies. The septa in the radiolucency give it a soap bubble or honeycomb appearance. Some ameloblastomas are unilocular. Some are associated with unerupted teeth (usually mandibular third molars) and, therefore, cannot be differentiated radiographically from dentigerous cysts. The teeth in the vicinity of the lesion may be tilted or moved bodily because of the generally slow growth rate of the tumor. Sometimes root resorption may appear in association with the growth of an ameloblastoma, but this is an uncommon phenomenon. An ameloblastoma infiltrates the surrounding intact bone before the destruction is visible on a radiograph. Therefore, pathologically, the lesion is much larger than its radiographic appearance. The local infiltration of surrounding bone gives the lesion its high recurrence rate, especially if treated conservatively by curettage instead of by marginal or block resection.

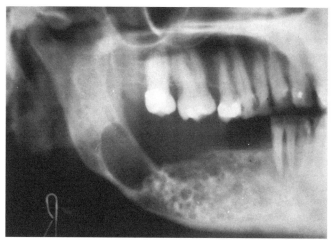

Figure 14–1

Ameloblastoma showing a large monolocular lesion with adjacent small multilocular spaces having a soap bubble appearance.

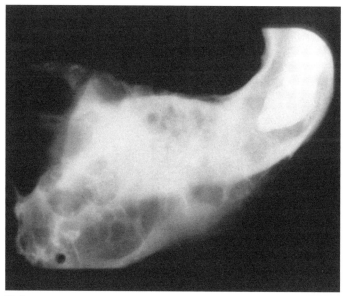

Figure 14–2

Surgical specimen of an ameloblastoma that shows a buccal cortical plate expansion and has a multilocular soap bubble appearance.

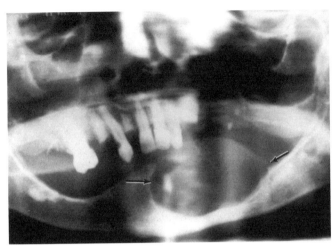

Figure 14–3
Unilocular ameloblastoma that shows an expansion into the oral cavity.

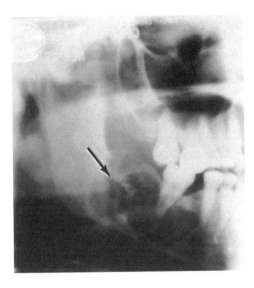

Figure 14–4
Multilocular ameloblastoma in the mandibular molar region.

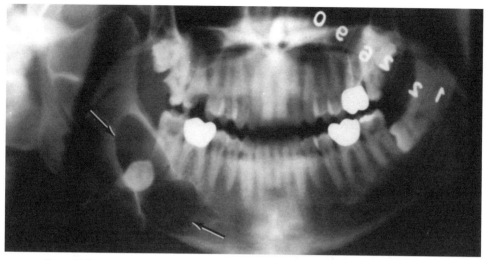

Figure 14–5

Ameloblastoma that resembles an odontogenic cyst (dentigerous cyst). A careful clinical and radiographic examination showed an expansion of the cortical bone.

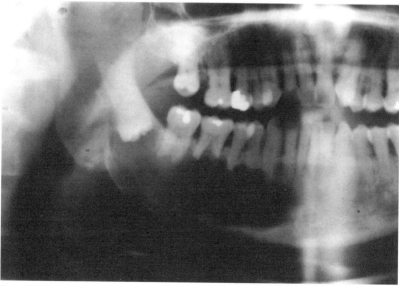

Figure 14–6

Ameloblastoma producing root resorption. Notice the evidence of expansion at the inferior border of the mandible. The lesion resembles a dentigerous cyst surrounding the crown of the impacted mandibular third molar.

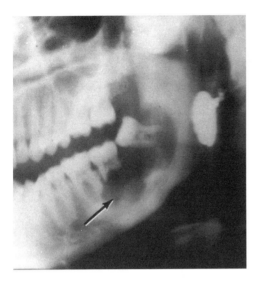

Figure 14–7
Ameloblastoma producing resorption of the roots of the second mandibular molar. The radiopaque object posterior to the ramus is an earring.

ODONTOGENIC ADENOMATOID TUMOR (ADENOAMELOBLASTOMA)

Odontogenic adenomatoid tumor, also known as adenomatoid odontogenic tumor, is a benign, encapsulated, painless, epithelial odontogenic neoplasm which grows by expansion and is usually associated with an unerupted tooth. The tumor is asymptomatic and small lesions are discovered incidentally on radiographic examination or when failure of tooth eruption is investigated. The swelling produced by a large lesion causes asymmetry. About 65 percent of the cases occur in the maxilla. The canine region is the most frequently involved area in both jaws. The mean age of patients is about 18 years. Females tend to be more commonly affected than males.

The radiographic appearance is that of a well-circumscribed unilocular lesion which may be completely radiolucent or may contain faint to dense radiopaque flecks of calcification. The radiolucency resembles a dentigerous cyst but envelopes most of the tooth rather than only the crown. Sometimes the radiolucency may occur without being associated with an unerupted tooth. As the tumor enlarges, it produces separation of roots or displacement of adjacent teeth.

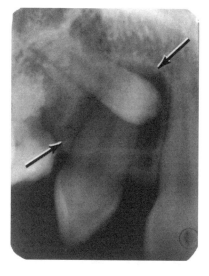

Figure 14–8

Odontogenic adenomatoid tumor resembles a dentigerous cyst and is associated with an impacted maxillary anterior tooth. The radiolucency must be differentiated from a normal follicular space and from other pericoronal lesions.

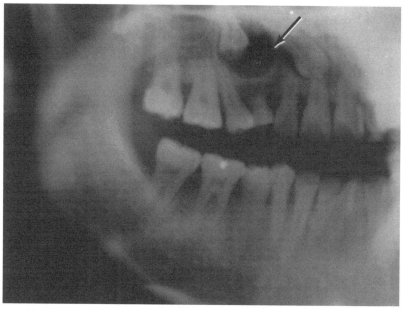

Figure 14–9

Odontogenic adenomatoid tumor associated with an impacted first premolar. The pericoronal radiolucency must be differentiated from other pericoronal lesions. A careful examination shows faint radiopaque flecks of calcification in the radiolucency.

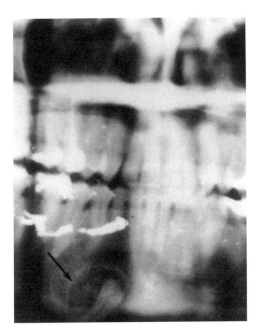

Figure 14–10

Odontogenic adenomatoid tumor showing multiple radiopaque foci (calcifications) pericoronal to the impacted mandibular permanent canine. The radiopaque line near the superior border of the mandible suggests that the patient had undergone sialography for an unrelated symptom.

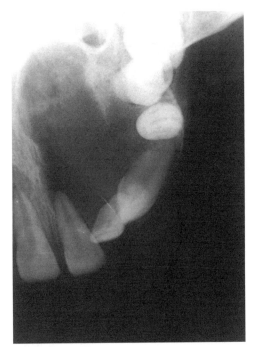

Figure 14–11

An occlusal projection showing an odontogenic adenomatoid tumor in the maxillary anterior region. The lesion can occur without being associated with an unerupted tooth. There is presence of a swelling in the canine region and divergence of the roots of the anterior teeth.

CALCIFYING EPITHELIAL ODONTOGENIC TUMOR (PINDBORG TUMOR)

Calcifying epithelial odontogenic tumor, also known as Pindborg tumor, is a rare lesion which behaves very much like an ameloblastoma. Jaw expansion or incidental observation on radiographs is the usual way in which this lesion is discovered. It is found in about the same age group as an ameloblastoma with a mean around 40 years. The tumor has a definite predilection for the mandible. Any site in the jaw may be affected but the premolar - molar areas are more susceptible. About 50 percent of the cases are associated with unerupted teeth. This slow-growing lesion is mainly asymptomatic but may sometimes produce a painless swelling over the involved region. It is locally aggressive, infiltrates the surrounding tissues like an ameloblastoma and is, therefore, more likely to recur after surgical treatment.

Radiographic appearance reveals a cyst-like area which may or may not be well-delineated. In half the number of cases, the appearance mimics that of a dentigerous cyst or even an ameloblastoma. Large lesions tend to be multilocular and may exhibit honeycomb appearance. As the lesion matures, the radiograph reveals a unilocular or multilocular cystic lesion with numerous scattered radiopaque flecks. Sometimes the roots of the teeth may be resorbed.

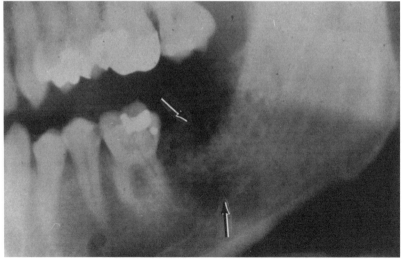

Figure 14–12
Calcifying epithelial odontogenic tumor involving the mandibular second and third molar region. Radiographically, the lesion shows a honeycomb appearance. (Courtesy Dr. J. Weir).

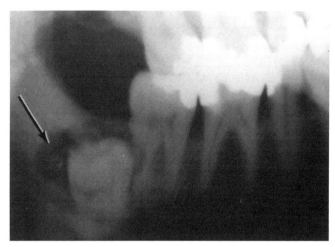

Figure 14–13

Calcifying epithelial odontogenic tumor (Pindborg tumor) involving an unerupted tooth. The well-delineated pericoronal radiolucency around the mandibular third molar contains numerous scattered radiopaque flecks of calcification.

AMELOBLASTIC FIBROMA

Ameloblastic fibroma is a mixed odontogenic tumor composed of odontogenic epithelium and mesenchyme. It occurs less frequently than an ameloblastoma. Its occurrence is during the period of tooth formation; that is, between the ages of 5 and 20 years whereas ameloblastomas generally occur in the fourth or fifth decade of life. Over 90 percent of the lesions are pericoronal and may be difficult to distinguish from dentigerous cysts. Unlike an ameloblastoma, this benign, painless lesion enlarges by slow expansion, bulging the cortical plates rather than eroding them. The lesion does not infiltrate the surrounding tissues, and therefore, does not recur when surgically treated. The site of occurrence is the same as that of an ameloblastoma: the mandibular premolar-molar area.

On a radiograph, the ameloblastic fibroma cannot be distinguished from a simple ameloblastoma. It is seen as an area of uniform radiolucency that has a smooth and well-defined border. The lesion may be either unilocular or multilocular. Frequently it is associated with an unerupted tooth which is often displaced to a significant distance and adjacent roots may be pushed apart by the tumor. Very often the lesion is pericoronal to a mandibular molar.

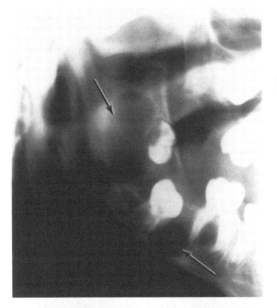

Figure 14–14
Ameloblastic fibroma associated with unerupted and displaced mandibular second and third molars. The lesion is pericoronal to the teeth which are in the formative stages.

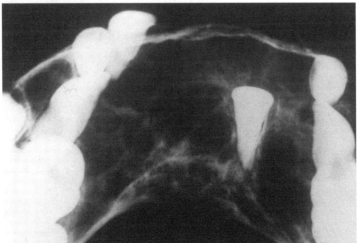

Figure 14–15
Ameloblastic fibroma showing a multilocular appearance and associated with an unerupted displaced incisor. There is expansion of the mandible. Although most ameloblastic fibromas occur in the mandibular premolar-molar areas, other sites may sometimes be affected as seen in this case. (Courtesy Dr. J. Weir).

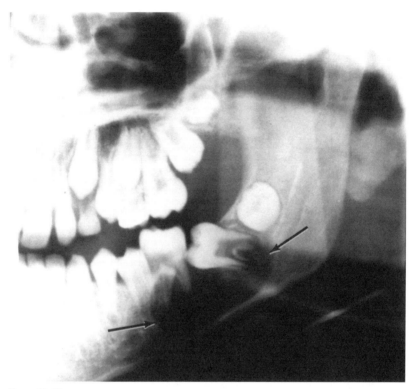

Figure 14–16
Ameloblastic fibroma associated with the mandibular molars.

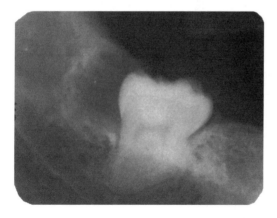

Figure 14–17
Ameloblastic fibroma growing superiorly and distally to the crown of the unerupted third molar. The lesion should be differentiated from other pericoronal lesions.

AMELOBLASTIC ODONTOMA

Ameloblastic odontoma is a rare clinical entity. It is characterized as an ameloblastoma with induction of mature dental tissues. It is essentially an ameloblastoma in which there is focal differentiation into an odontoma. An ameloblastic odontoma may be radiographically indistinguishable from a complex odontoma. There is a tendency for the radiopaque mass to occupy a relatively smaller proportion of the radiolucency than in the case of an odontoma. The lesion may displace the associated tooth.

AMELOBLASTIC FIBRO-ODONTOMA

Ameloblastic fibro-odontoma is a separate entity from ameloblastic odontoma. Ameloblastic fibro-odontoma is a lesion that consists of an ameloblastic fibroma and an odontoma. According to the maturation theory, this lesion represents an ameloblastic fibroma which matures into an ameloblastic fibro-odontoma. Some investigators state that if an ameloblastic fibroma is left undisturbed for a long time, it would ultimately mature completely into a complex composite odontoma. Most examples have been found in children, the average age being 12 years. The mandible has a slightly higher incidence of ameloblastic fibro-odontoma than the maxilla. The most common site affected is the premolar-molar region.

Radiographically, most ameloblastic fibro-odontomas are associated with crowns of impacted teeth. The lesions are well-demarcated. They may be unilocular or multilocular radiolucencies containing multiple radiopaque foci with irregular configurations. Recurrence is essentially non-existent because the lesion enucleates with relative ease from the bony defect.

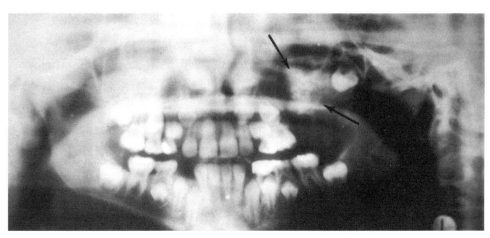

Figure 14–18

Ameloblastic fibro-odontoma is pericoronal to the impacted maxillary third molar and involves the maxillary sinus.

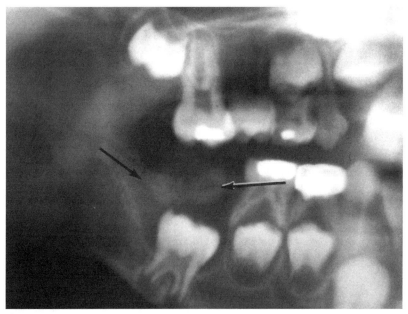

Figure 14–19

Ameloblastic fibro-odontoma located superior to the crown of an erupting mandibular permanent first molar in a 6-year-old child.

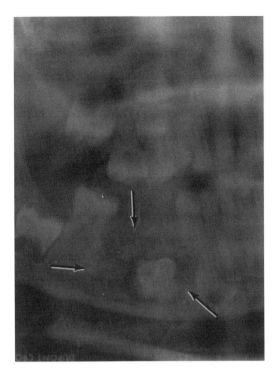

Figure 14-20
Ameloblastic fibro-
odontoma associated
with the crown of an
unerupted molar in a
child.

ODONTOMA
(HAMARTOMA)

1) Compound composite odontoma. It is a collection of small radiopaque masses, some or all of which may be tooth-like. The numbers vary from two to several dozen. These unerupted tooth-like masses have a tendency to occur in the anterior segments of the jaws with a somewhat greater incidence in the maxilla. A compound odontoma is formed by an exuberant growth of the dental lamina or by proliferation of an enamel organ into a number of small enamel organs. Microscopic sections show multiple tooth-like structures complete with enamel matrix, dentin and a central pulp chamber. The toothlets are so closely packed together that they appear to be one mass. The lesion is surrounded by a radiolucent line and bounded by a radiopaque border.

2) Complex composite odontoma. It is a mass of unorganized dental tissues. The enamel, dentin, cementum and pulp are arranged in a haphazard form. The conglomerate calcified mass has no resemblance to a normal tooth. It is a self-limiting lesion that tends to occur in the posterior segments of the jaws with a somewhat greater incidence in the mandible. Depending on whether the lesion arises from a normal tooth follicle or a supernumerary tooth follicle, there might or might not be a missing tooth. On a radiograph, the radiopaque mass may be of varying densities. Often, an unerupted tooth is associated with the mass. The lesion may be surrounded by a radiolucent line and bounded by a radiopaque border.

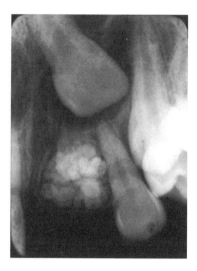

Figure 14–21
Compound odontoma showing small radiopaque masses preventing eruption of the central incisor.

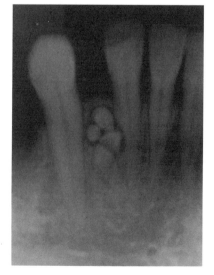

Figure 14–22
Compound odontoma showing small toothlets. The lesion is surrounded by a radiolucent line.

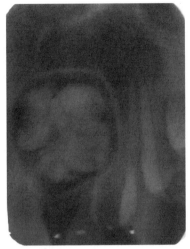

Figure 14–23
Compound odontoma exhibiting a prominent peripheral radiolucency bordered by a radiopaque line.

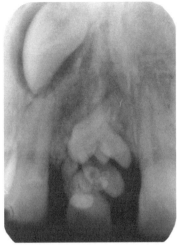

Figure 14–24
Compound odontoma consisting of small toothlets.

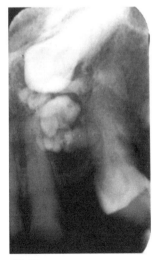

Figure 14–25
Compound odontoma consisting of small toothlets.

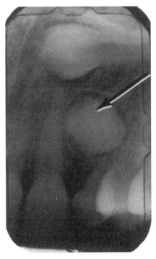

Figure 14–26
Complex odontoma obstructing the permanent canine from erupting. The lesion is surrounded by a radiolucent periphery. There is retention of the deciduous canine.

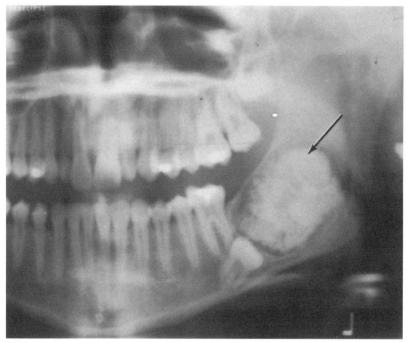

Figure 14–27
Complex odontoma in the mandibular third molar and ramus region. A radiolucent line surrounds the lesion.

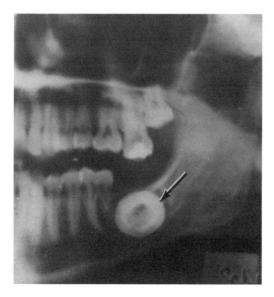

Figure 14–28
Complex odontoma developed from the mandibular second molar.

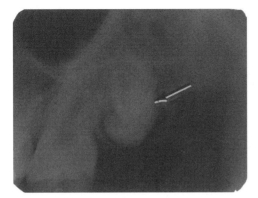

Figure 14–29
Complex odontoma developed from the maxillary third molar.

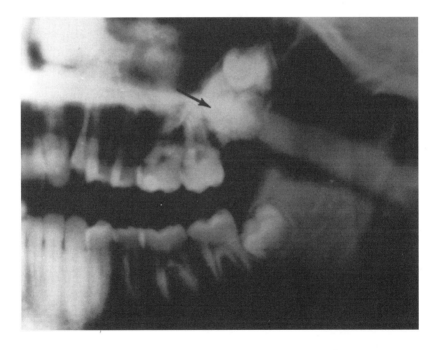

Figure 14–30
Complex odontoma in the maxillary tuberosity and associated with the crown of the unerupted maxillary third molar.

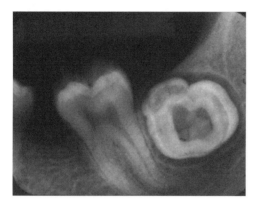

Figure 14–31
Complex odontoma
developing from the
mandibular third molar.

ODONTOGENIC MYXOMA
(ODONTOGENIC FIBROMYXOMA, MYXOFIBROMA)

The odontogenic myxoma originates from the mesenchymal portions of the tooth bud, probably from the dental papilla. When relatively large amounts of collagen are evident, the term myxofibroma may be used to designate this entity. That the tumor is odontogenic seems quite plausible, since apparently it is not found in bones outside the facial skeleton. It occurs almost exclusively in the tooth-bearing regions of the jaws and the myxomatous tissue histologically resembles the stellate reticulum found in developing teeth. The tumor is asymptomatic although some patients complain of pain. It occurs in individuals between the ages of 10 and 30 years. It has been stated that it is unusual to find it in persons younger than 10 years or older than 50 years. When it grows to a large size, it causes cortical expansion rather than perforation of the cortical bone. The swelling may be large enough to produce facial asymmetry. Some cases are associated with impacted teeth. The body and posterior portion of the mandible are the favored sites. Maxillary myxomas may perforate and invade the antrum.

On a radiograph, the lesion appears as a radiolucency containing extremely delicate septa, giving it a multilocular or honeycomb appearance similar to an ameloblastoma, a giant cell granuloma, and a fibrous dysplasia. The multilocular compartments differ from other lesions in that they tend to be angular and may be separated by straight septa that form square, rectangular, or triangular spaces. The margins of the lesion are poorly defined. The roots of adjoining teeth may be displaced. In some instances, the lesion may be unilocular, particularly if it arises from the part of the follicle that persists in the pericoronal region of an unerupted tooth. Although myxomas are benign, they are locally invasive and, therefore, have a high recurrence rate following attempts at curettage. The overall prognosis for this lesion, however, is good.

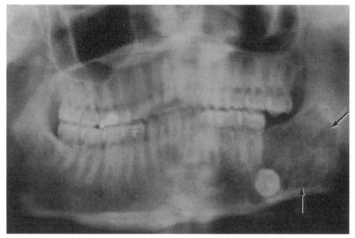

Figure 14–32
Odontogenic fibromyxoma of the left mandible showing a honeycomb expansible lesion associated with an impacted tooth.

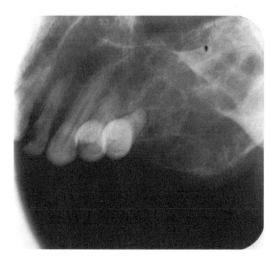

Figure 14–33
Odontogenic myxoma exhibiting the characteristic multilocular appearnce with straight septa forming squares, rectangles and triangles.

ODONTOGENIC FIBROMA

Central odontogenic fibroma is an infrequent lesion and, therefore, very little is known about it. This rare lesion is regarded as the bony counterpart to the peripheral odontogenic fibroma. It arises from the mesenchymal components of a tooth germ, either the dental follicle, dental papilla, or the periodontal ligament. The mandible may be the most common location for this tumor. This benign, painless, slow-growing, asymptomatic tumor produces cortical expansion of the jawbone. On a radiograph, the lesion exhibits either a unilocular or a multilocular radiolucency similar to that of an ameloblastoma. The lesion shows little tendency to recur after curettage.

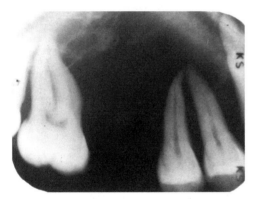

Figure 14–34
Odontogenic fibroma involving the premolar-molar region.

CEMENTIFYING FIBROMA (OSSIFYING FIBROMA, CEMENTO-OSSIFYING FIBROMA)

Cementifying fibroma or ossifying fibroma is a benign fibro-osseous lesion of periodontal ligament origin. Clinically, this mesenchymal odontogenic neoplasm manifests as a painless enlargement with cortical expansion, resulting in displacement of teeth or divergence of roots. The most common sites are the tooth-bearing areas of the mandible. Most cases are seen in young to middle-aged adults.

On a radiograph, the morphology of the lesion depends on the stage of tumor development. In the first stage, the lesion is a unilocular, well-circumscribed radiolucency and may be mistaken for a cyst. In the second stage, the radiolucency shows multiple small radiopaque foci of calcified masses. In the final stage, the calcified masses coalesce to form a solid radiopacity with a peripheral radiolucent rim. The teeth adjacent to the tumor are vital and may be displaced or their roots may be diverged. The prognosis is good since most cementifying fibromas respond well to enucleation or curettage. See also Chapter 7 (Apical Lesions).

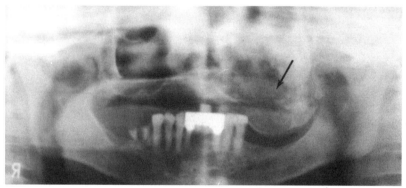

Figure 14–35
Cementifying fibroma (ossifying fibroma) exhibiting foci of calcified masses and producing expansion of the left maxillary sinus. A similar appearance may sometimes be seen in fibrous dysplasia.

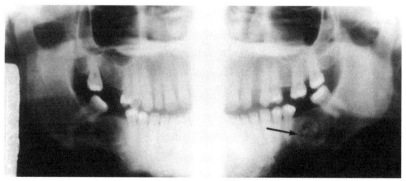

Figure 14–36
Cementifying fibroma (ossifying fibroma) showing calcification in the radiolucency located between the mandibular left second premolar and third molar.

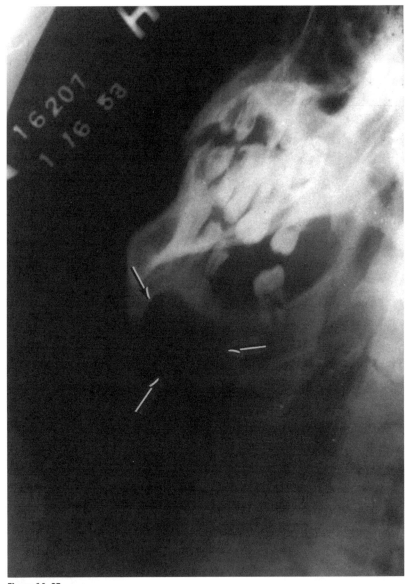

Figure 14–37
Ossifying fibroma in the radiolucent stage showing expansion of the cortical bone of the mandible.

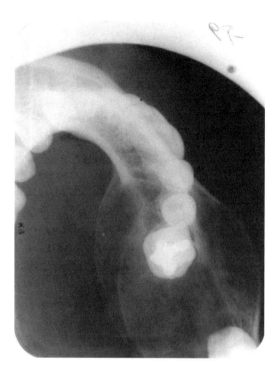

Figure 14–38
Ossifying fibroma exhibiting radiopaque foci of calcified material. The lesion shows buccal and lingual expansion of cortical bone.

CEMENTOBLASTOMA

Cementoblastoma is a benign mesenchymal odontogenic neoplasm that forms a large bulbous mass of cementum on the roots of a tooth. It is also known as a true cementoma. It occurs predominantly in the second and third decades, typically before 25 years of age. It arises in association with the apex or apices of a mandibular molar or premolar tooth, usually the first mandibular molar. The tooth remains vital and its position is not affected. Usually there are no symptoms but when the lesion is large, there may be slight expansion of the cortical plates.

On a radiograph, the morphology of the lesion depends on the stage of development, similar to the three stages of cementifying fibroma. The lesion, when discovered, is usually in the third stage consisting of a discrete radiopaque mass with a thin radiolucent border and attached to the root of the affected tooth. This prognosis is good after extraction of the involved tooth and excision of the mass. See also Chapter 7 (Apical Lesions).

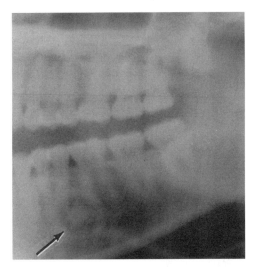

Figure 14–39

Cementoblastoma in the third stage consisting of a radiopaque mass with a radiolucent border and attached to the apices of the mandibular second premolar and first molar. The teeth are vital.

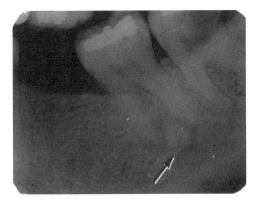

Figure 14–40

Cementoblastoma consisting of a radiopaque mass with a radiolucent border and attached to the apices of the mandibular second molar. The involved tooth is vital.

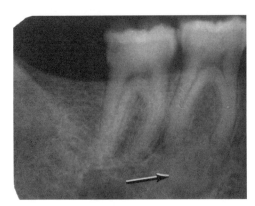

Figure 14–41

Cementoblastoma at the root apices of the mandibular first molar. The involved tooth is vital.

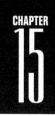

CHAPTER 15

NONODONTOGENIC BENIGN TUMORS OF THE JAWS

Exostoses and Tori

Osteoma

Osteoid Osteoma

Central Hemangioma

Arteriovenous Fistula

Neurogenic Tumors (neurilemmoma, neurofibroma)

Traumatic Neuroma

Chondroma

TUMOR-LIKE AND REACTIVE LESIONS

Central Giant Cell Granuloma

Fibrous Dysplasia

Histiocytosis X

EXOSTOSES AND TORI

Exostoses and tori are localized peripheral overgrowths of bone due to some unknown cause. Although etiology is unknown, a hereditary basis is suspected. They are prevalent in certain populations; the highest incidence is in Eskimos, American Indians, and Asians. They occur on any surface of the jaw bones. When a bony protuberance occurs in the midline of the palate, it is called a torus palatinus; when it occurs on the lingual surface of the mandible, it is called a torus mandibularis. When multiple small nodular protuberances appear on the buccal surfaces of the alveolar bone, they are called exostoses. The palatal torus occurs in about 25 percent of the U. S. population and is twice as prevalent in females than in males. The mandibular torus occurs in about 7 percent of the U.S. population and has no predilection to a specific sex. Very small exostoses and tori consist entirely of compact bone but when large and nodular, the center consists of cancellous bone which is surrounded by compact bone. They vary in size from a slight elevation to a large protuberance.

Exostoses and tori are neither of pathological nor of clinical significance except that they interfere with normal speech and other functions. They also interfere with the preparation and insertion of prosthetic appliances, in which case surgical removal of the exostosis or torus may be contemplated. On a radiograph, exostoses and tori appear as well-defined round or oval radiopacities superimposed on the roots of teeth. If the radiopacities are at the apical ends of the roots, they may be confused with osteosclerosis. Unlike osteosclerosis, torus mandibularis occurs almost always bilaterally.

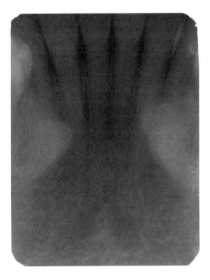

Figure 15–1
Mandibular tori seen bilaterally.

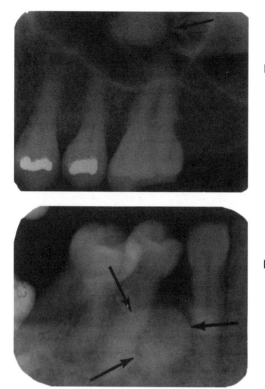

Figure 15–2
Torus palatinus as seen on a periapical film.

Figure 15–3
Mandibular torus

OSTEOMA

Osteoma is a benign tumor of bone which occurs most commonly on the skull and jaw bones. It also occurs on long bones as an osteochondroma. It is composed primarily of cortical bone or cancellous bone, or a combination of cortical and cancellous bones. The bony-hard discrete mass extends from the cortex and produces asymmetry of the jaw. Osteomas can also occur in maxillary and frontoethmoidal sinuses. Multiple osteomas of the jaws as well as of long bones and skull are a characteristic manifestation of Gardner's syndrome. In Gardner's syndrome, the patient has multiple osteomas, multiple polyps of the large intestine, multiple epidermoid cysts, desmoid (fibrous) tumors of skin, and impacted supernumerary and permanent teeth. On a radiograph, an osteoma presents a radiopaque mass projecting from the surface of bone.

When composed of compact bone it is a completely opaque mass, but when composed of cancellous bone it shows evidence of internal trabecular structure.

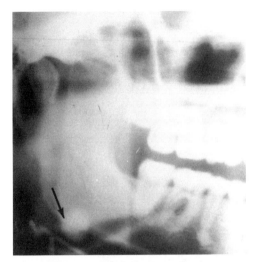

Figure 15–4
Osteoma of the compact bone arising from the mandibular cortex. It has to be differentiated from a calcified lymph node and a sialolith because of their similar radiographic appearance.

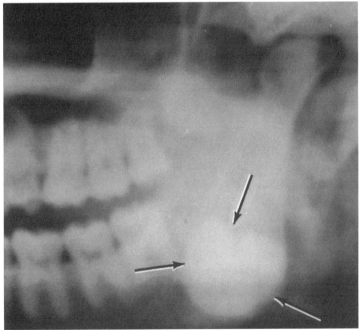

Figure 15–5
Osteoma arising from the angle of the mandible.

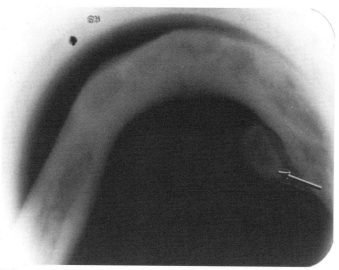

Figure 15–6

Osteoma of the mandible which is attached by a pedicle and could be palpated clinically. This osteoma consists of a combination of cortical and cancellous bones. The osteoma should be differentiated from a sialolith.

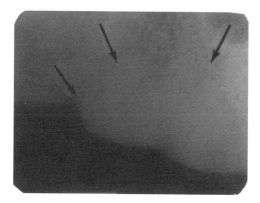

Figure 15–7

Osteoma arising from the edentulous alveolar bone. The osteoma is of compact bone.

OSTEOID OSTEOMA

Osteoid osteoma is a variation of an osteoma and rarely occurs in the jaws. It occurs most commonly in the femur and tibia. This benign tumor is found in young persons under the age of 30. It occurs in or near the cortex and may produce swelling of overlying soft tissue. There is intense pain which is out of proportion to the size of the lesion. The radiographic appearance is very characteristic and shows a radiopaque nidus of osteoid tissue containing trabeculae. The osteoid tissue is surrounded by a diffuse and irregular radiolucency of vascular connective tissue which is surrounded by a rim of sclerotic bone. The radiographic appearance is sometimes confused with that of chronic suppurative osteomyelitis. Subperiosteal thickening may take place with the formation of new bone under the periosteum. There is no recurrence if the lesion is completely excised.

Osteoid osteoma bears considerable clinical, radiographic, and histologic similarity to a benign tumor called osteoblastoma. Many experts, in fact, regard the two lesions as identical. Classically, the distinction rests primarily on the size of the lesion: osteoid osteoma is under 2 cm, and osteoblastoma is larger than 2 cm.

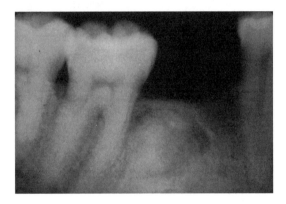

Figure 15–8
Osteoid osteoma in the region between the premolar and molar teeth.

CENTRAL HEMANGIOMA

Central hemangioma is a benign vascular neoplasm within bone which produces a proliferation of blood vessels. It occurs more often in the vertebrae and skull but rarely in the jaws. The posterior region of the mandible is the most frequent site of occurrence. The tumor is seen in children and teenagers; females are affected twice as often as males. The lesion produces a hard, nontender, slow-growing swelling. The teeth in the vicinity of the tumor may be loosened and bleeding may occur from the gingiva around the necks of the affected teeth. The teeth have increased hypermobility and may exhibit a pumping action such that when depressed in an apical direction, the teeth rapidly resume their original position. The lesion may pulsate and a bruit may be detected on auscultation. Some hemangiomas may be present without any sign or symptom.

The radiographic appearance may take many forms; in most instances it is that of a cyst having a well-defined radiolucency surrounded by a sclerotic border. Sometimes the lesion shows the classic multilocular radiolucency called honeycomb or soap bubble appearance. The roots of the teeth may be resorbed. The cortical region may be thinned and expanded. The differential diagnosis of a central hemangioma is difficult because of its multiple radiographic appearances. Sometimes radiopaque phleboliths may be visible in the radiolucency. If an angiogram is taken, it will demonstrate the increased vascular supply to the lesion. A central hemangioma is a great surgical risk (including tooth extraction) since bleeding is difficult to control. Therefore, before surgery, the patient must be prepared for emergency blood transfusion and ligation of the carotids. Sometimes partial maxillectomy and mandibulectomy may be necessary. After adequate removal of the tumor, the prognosis is good because the lesion does not recur and is not malignant.

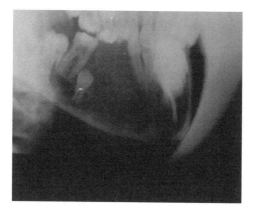

Figure 15–9
Central hemangioma involving the entire body of the mandible and showing a coarse trabecular pattern (Courtesy Dr. A. Wuehrmann and Dr. L. Manson-Hing).

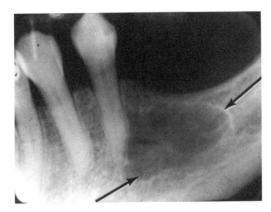

Figure 15–10
Central hemangioma showing a well-circumscribed cavity.

ARTERIOVENOUS FISTULA (ARTERIOVENOUS SHUNT OR MALFORMATION)

Arteriovenous fistula is a direct communication between an artery and a vein, bypassing the intervening capillaries. It can occur in soft tissue or in bone as a result of trauma or a developmental anomaly. There may or may not be the presence of a swelling. Aspiration of the involved site will produce blood. Arteriovenous fistulae may be confused with hemangiomas. On a radiograph, the lesion may be unilocular or multilocular. The most characteristic location for its occurrence is the ramus-retromolar area of the mandible involving the mandibular canal. Sometimes phleboliths may occur in the lesion. An angiogram may be necessary to show the vascular nature of the lesion.

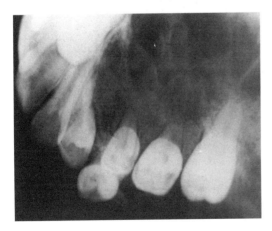

Figure 15–11
Arteriovenous fistula involving the whole palate (Courtesy Dr. John Coryn).

Neurogenic Tumors

Neurogenic tumors are rare benign intraosseous nerve tumors which occur mostly in the body and ramus of the mandible. This is explained by the fact that the mandibular canal conveys a large neurovascular bundle for a longer distance than does any other bony canal. These tumors arise from the nerve sheaths as well as from the nerve fibers in combination with their supporting tissues.

NEURILEMMOMA (SCHWANNOMA)

Although neurilemmoma is a rare tumor, it is the most common of the neurogenic tumors. It arises from the Schwann's cells which make up the inner layer covering the peripheral nerves. This slow-growing encapsulated benign tumor occurs at any age and may cause expansion and perforation of the cortical plates with subsequent soft tissue swelling. The soft tissue nodular mass is usually painless although pain may occur in rare instances. The tongue is the favored location, although lesions have been described in the palate, floor of the mouth, buccal mucosa, gingiva, lips, vestibule, and jaws. Bony lesions show a radiographic finding of a radiolucent area of bone distal to the mental foramen, surrounded by a well-defined radiopaque border similar to that of a cyst. Sometimes the lesion may be multilocular. The lesion has an intimate relationship with the mandibular canal. Like all nerve tumors, the neurilemmoma is not responsive to x-radiation therapy. Therefore, surgical excision is the treatment of choice, especially since it is encapsulated (unlike neurofibroma which is nonencapsulated). For extensive bony lesions, curettage or resection should be performed.

NEUROFIBROMA

Neurofibroma is a benign slow-growing tumor composed of components from the peripheral nerves (including the axons) and from the connective tissue of the sheath of Schwann. Although the tumor is not common, it is by no means a clinical rarity. It can occur in soft tissue and/or in bone. Neurofibromas may appear as solitary lesions or as

313

multiple lesions as part of von Recklinghausen's disease (syndrome neurofibromatosis). Neurofibroma occurs at any age but is usually found in young patients and has a high potential for malignant change. The solitary neurofibroma is asymptomatic and occurs on the tongue, buccal mucosa, and vestibule. The swelling is firm on palpation and may perforate the cortex. The central (bony) lesion associated with a mandibular nerve is most likely to produce pain and paresthesia. On a radiograph, a central neurofibroma of the inferior dental nerve appears as a fusiform enlargement of the canal. The margins of the lesion may or may not be sharply defined. The tumor is not sensitive to x-radiation therapy. The syndrome of von Recklinghausen's neurofibromatosis includes multiple neurofibromas on the skin, cutaneous café-au-lait spots (especially diagnostic when located in the axilla), bone deformities and neurologic abnormalities.

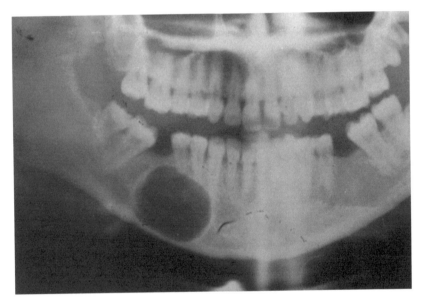

Figure 15–12
Neurilemmoma (schwannoma) involving the mandibular canal and the mentalforamen. The lesion has a well-defined radiopaque border (Courtesy Dr. Doug Damm).

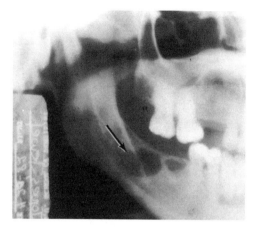

Figure 15–13
Neurofibroma of the inferior dental nerve demonstrating a multilocular form.

TRAUMATIC NEUROMA
(AMPUTATION NEUROMA, NEUROMA)

Traumatic neuroma is not a true tumor but is a proliferation produced by a damaged or severed nerve trunk. The trauma to the nerve is caused by tooth extraction, local anesthetic injection, jaw fracture, soft tissue trauma, ill-fitting denture or accident. The traumatized nerve segments proliferate in an attempt to regenerate and re-establish innervation. When these nerve elements get entangled and trapped in the developing scar tissue, they form a composite mass of fibrous tissue and disorganized nerve at the site of injury. This tumor of neural elements and scar tissue is nonencapsulated. Unlike neurilemmoma and neurofibroma, neuralgic pain is experienced locally and in distant parts. The type of pain varies from one patient to another and ranges from occasional tenderness to constant severe pain.

In the oral cavity, the mental foramen is the most common site of occurrence, presumably arising following tooth extraction with damage to the mental nerve. Other common sites are alveolar ridge, lips and tongue where the small nodules of traumatic neuroma are visible. In the soft tissues, the nodule of traumatic neuroma is of normal color, firm and sessile. Traumatic neuroma should be included in a clinical differential diagnosis of any small mass that is spontaneously painful or painful when compressed. The bony lesion shows a discrete radiolucency. The lesion should be surgically excised along with the obstructing agent. Some cases may experience continued pain despite the absence of a lesion.

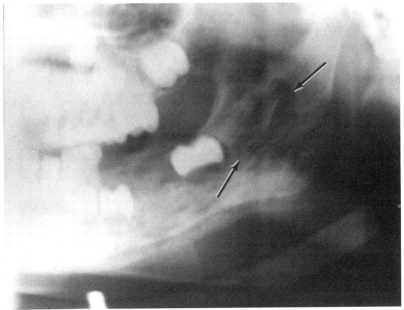

Figure 15–14
Traumatic neuroma associated with a fracture of the ramus. Note the fracture extending from the posterior border of the ramus.

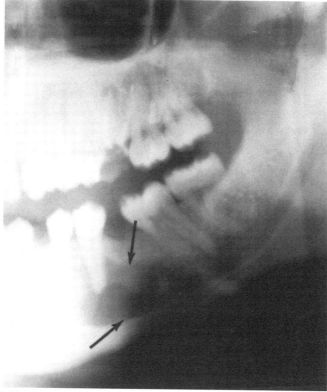

Figure 15–15

Traumatic neuroma associated with the extraction site of the mandibular first molar. Note the bulbous enlargement of the mandibular canal due to increased growth.

CHONDROMA

Chondroma is a central benign cartilaginous tumor. Although it is common in other parts of the body, it is exceedingly rare in the jaws. The anterior portion of the maxilla, condyle and coronoid process are the most commonly involved. A chondroma is a painless, slow-growing tumor producing destruction and exfoliation of teeth. Tumors that involve condyle and coronoid process may affect mandibular function. On a radiograph, the tumor appears as cyst-like radiolucencies; some are sclerotic. The borders are usually ill-defined. Irregular calcifications may occur with the radiolucencies and then it is called an osteochondroma. Roots of the involved teeth may be resorbed. A chondrosarcoma can develop from a pre-existing chondroma.

CENTRAL GIANT CELL GRANULOMA

Central giant cell granuloma is a fairly common lesion which occurs almost exclusively in the jawbones; the mandible is more frequently affected than the maxilla (3:1 ratio). The lesion occurs in the first three decades of life prior to 30 years of age. Its etiology is unknown. Investigators regard the lesion as either a reparative response or a benign nonodontogenic tumor or a developmental anomaly related closely to the aneurysmal bone cyst. The lesion occurs exclusively in the tooth-bearing areas of the jaws anterior to the molar teeth. When located near the anterior teeth, it is one of the few intrabony jaw lesions to cross the midline. A small lesion is detected incidentally on radiographic examination for an unrelated purpose. A large lesion is detected in the investigation of an asymptomatic localized expansion of a jawbone producing facial asymmetry.

Radiographic appearance is classically that of a multilocular radiolucency with discrete scalloped borders. Of the different types of multilocular lesions, the central giant cell granuloma is the single most common multilocular lesion. A few central giant cell granulomas appear as unilocular radiolucencies. The margins of the lesion may be either well-defined or poorly defined. Teeth may be displaced in cases of jaw expansion. In some cases, the central type of giant cell granuloma may be associated with the peripheral type. Since the histologic features of the giant cell granuloma are indistinguishable from those of a brown tumor of hyperparathyroidism, it is prudent to evaluate any patient with a central giant cell granuloma for the possibility of hyperparathyroidism. Treatment consists of conservative surgical removal by curettage. The prognosis is excellent with only rare recurrences.

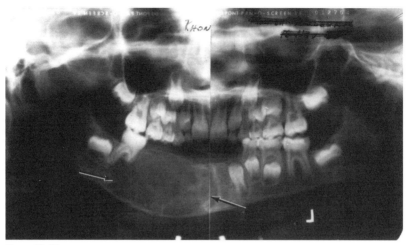

Figure 15–16
Central giant cell granuloma exhibiting a multilocular radiolucency with a localized expansion of the jawbone.

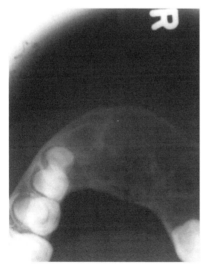

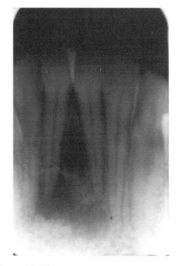

Figure 15–17
Central giant cell granuloma shows jaw expansion on an occlusal projection. The multilocular lesion crosses the midline of the mandible.

Figure 15–18
Central giant cell granuloma in the midline region of the mandible.

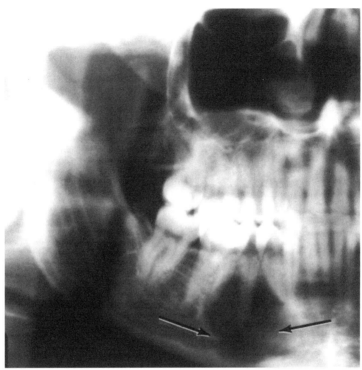

Figure 15–19
Central giant cell granuloma exhibiting a unilocular radiolucency with well-defined margins in the mandibular premolar region.

FIBROUS DYSPLASIA

Fibrous dysplasia is a benign fibro-osseous lesion in which normal medullary bone is gradually replaced by an abnormal fibrous connective tissue proliferation that contains foci of irregularly shaped trabeculae of immature bone. Microscopic examination shows these trabeculae to resemble written Chinese characters. Fibrous dysplasia has some features of a metabolic condition and some features of a neoplastic condition. The lesion begins before puberty but is discovered later on. Fibrous dysplasia presents three clinical forms: monostotic (occurs in a single bone), polyostotic (occurs in many bones), and Albright's syndrome. Albright's syndrome consists of polyostotic fibrous dysplasia, café-au-lait spots on skin (skin pigmentation), and precocious sexual development. Fibrous dysplasia may affect any bone in the skeleton but most often affects the skull and facial bones, or ribs. Monostotic fibrous dysplasia is much more common than the polyostotic form. A painless, slow enlargement of the affected bone produces facial asymmetry. The swelling is bony hard to palpation. The maxilla is more often involved than the mandible.

On a radiograph, the lesion is seldom well-defined; it tends to blend imperceptibly into adjacent normal bone. The radiographic appearance varies, depending on its stage of maturity. In the early (osteolytic) stage, the lesion appears as a radiolucency; in the intermediate stage, it appears as a ground glass or orange peel appearance; in the final (mature) stage, it appears as a radiopacity. Conservative osseous contouring for cosmetic correction should be delayed until after the cessation of growth of the skeleton and of the lesion.

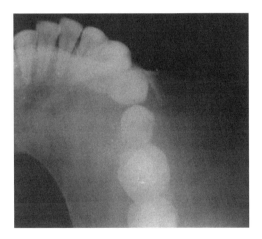

Figure 15–20
Fibrous dysplasia presenting a ground glass appearance and a unilateral expansion of the mandible.

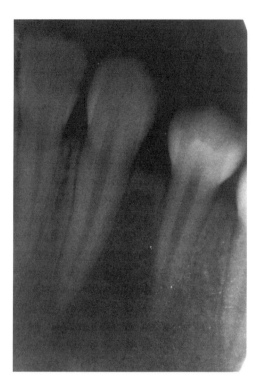

Figure 15–21
Fibrous dysplasia presenting a ground glass appearance.

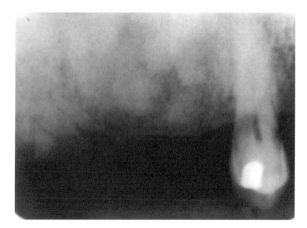

Figure 15–22
Fibrous dysplasia in the mature stage presenting a radiopaque image. The affected region is expanded.

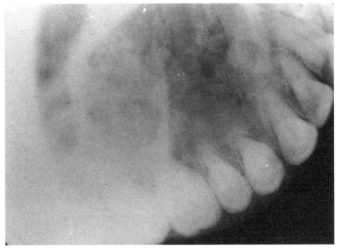

Figure 15–23
Fibrous dysplasia of the maxilla showing a mixed appearance of radiopacities and radiolucencies.

HISTIOCYTOSIS X
(RETICULOENDOTHELIOSIS, LANGERHANS' CELL GRANULOMATOSIS)

Histiocytosis X is a group of reticuloendothelial diseases that are not well understood; the etiology and pathogenesis are unknown. It acts like a metabolic and a neoplastic disease. The disease is characterized by a proliferation of differentiated histiocyte-like cells. The three entities making up this group are: Letterer-Siwe disease, Hand-Schüller-Christian disease, and eosinophilic granuloma. Histiocytosis X affects the reticuloendothelium organs such as the spleen, liver (hepatosplenomegaly), lymph nodes, bone marrow, and may infiltrate mucosa, skin or viscera. The jaws and oral soft tissues are involved in 20 percent of the cases and may be the only sites of the disease. The posterior region of the mandible is the most commonly involved site and may sometimes be associated with mild, dull pain. The radiographic appearance of teeth is that of "floating in air".

Letterer-Siwe disease occurs in the first three years of life. The disease often starts with a skin rash, persistent low-grade fever, malaise, and irritability. Other findings include hepatosplenomegaly, lymphadenopathy and anemia. In the oral cavity ulcerations may be present, as well as loss of alveolar bone. Severe cases usually result in death.

Hand-Schüller-Christian disease occurs in childhood between ages 3 to 10 years. In 10 percent of reported cases, the three classic signs are observed: bone lesions, diabetes insipidus (due to involvement of pituitary gland), and exophthalmos. The one or more punched-out radiolucent bone lesions of the skull are similar to the land and sea areas seen on a map, and hence are called a geographic skull. In the oral cavity there is severe loss of alveolar bone, which may resemble a common periodontal disease. Also, the oral soft-tissues may be involved.

Eosinophilic granuloma is believed to be a variant of Hand-Schüller-Christian disease and occurs in adolescents and young adults. It is a localized form of histiocytosis X. The skull and the jaws are both affected. The jaw lesions may be solitary or multiple radiolucencies and characteristically destroy the periodontal bone support of one or more teeth, especially in the posterior areas, resulting in "floating teeth."

Letterer-Siwe and Hand-Schüller-Christian diseases are treated by aggressive chemotherapy and radiotherapy similar to that used in leukemia. The prognosis of these two diseases is poor and often is fatal. Eosinophilic granuloma is usually treated by surgical curettage although radiotherapy is also effective. The prognosis of eosinophilic granuloma is good because there is only local destruction of tissue.

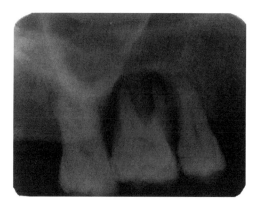

Figure 15–24
Eosinophilic granuloma (histiocytosis X) destroying the periodontal bone around the roots of the maxillary first molar and giving the appearance of a "floating tooth".

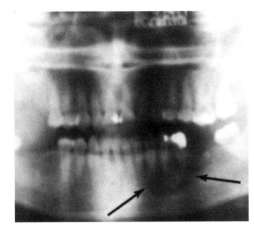

Figure 15–25
Eosinophilic granuloma destroying the bone around the mandibular left premolars and canine.

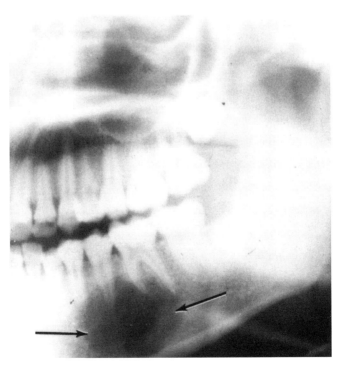

Figure 15–26
Eosinophilic granuloma in the apical region of the mandibular premolars and first molar.

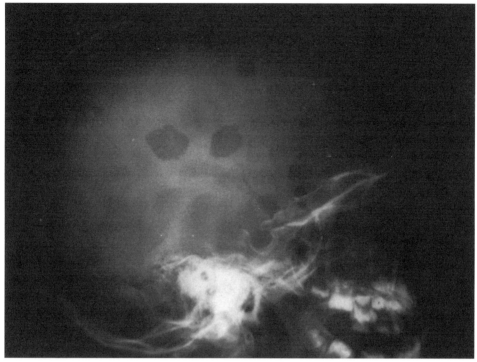

Figure 15–27

Hand-Schüller-Christian disease (histiocytosis X) showing multiple radiolucent skull lesions giving the appearance of a geographic skull.

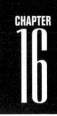

MALIGNANT TUMORS OF THE JAWS

Squamous cell carcinoma

Metastatic carcinoma

Sarcomas

Leukemia

Multiple myeloma

Malignant lymphomas

Burkitt's lymphoma

SQUAMOUS CELL CARCINOMA

Squamous cell carcinoma is a malignant tumor of epithelial origin. In the oral cavity, it arises from the oral mucosa. Most of the cases arise peripherally and some may invade the jaw bones, especially those that originate on or near the crest of the alveolar ridges and the posterior hard palate. In rare instances they may arise within the jaw bones (central type) from the epithelial cells of the dental lamina. Osseous involvement is seen most frequently in the mandibular third molar region. Carcinomas cause loosening or exfoliation of teeth. Squamous cell carcinoma spreads by direct extension into surrounding structures as well as by metastases through lymphatic channels. Thus, the lymph nodes involved in the metastatic spread of the lesion are enlarged, painless, very firm, immovable, and frequently matted together. These lymph nodes are in contrast to those of benign lymphadenitis (caused by infection) in which the nodes are enlarged, painful, firm, freely movable, and discrete.

On a radiograph, the erosion of the alveolar bone is seen as a radiolucent destructive lesion with ill-defined irregular margins. Radiographic appearances often simulate periodontal disease or periapical infection. The local destruction of bone produces the "teeth floating in space" appearance similar to that of histiocytosis X.

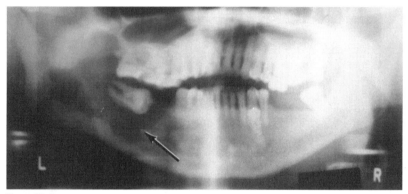

Figure 16–1

Squamous cell carcinoma producing destruction of bone around the left mandibular molar giving it a "tooth floating in space" appearance. Notice the diffuse and irregular borders of the lesion.

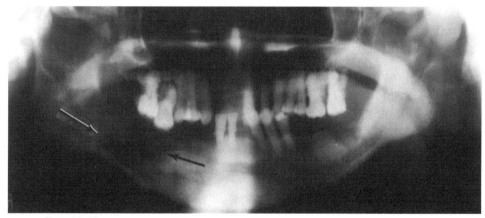

Figure 16–2A

Squamous cell carcinoma shows bone destruction in the mandibular right molar region.

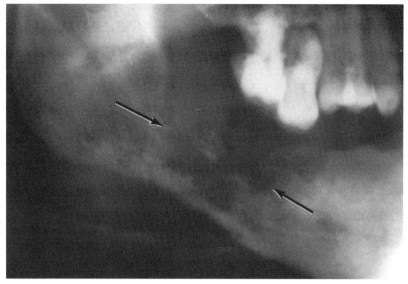

Figure 16–2B

Close-up of illustration. Squamous cell carcinoma of the alveolar ridge and surrounding mandibular bone. Notice the diffuse and irregular borders of the lesion.

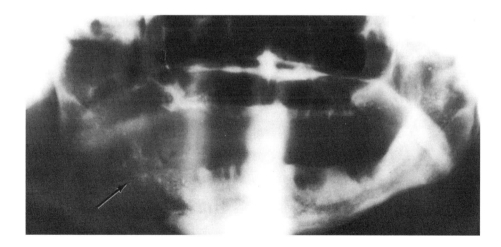

Figure 16–2C

The same squamous cell carcinoma after extraction of all the teeth. The radiograph was taken one month later and shows extensive bone destuction.

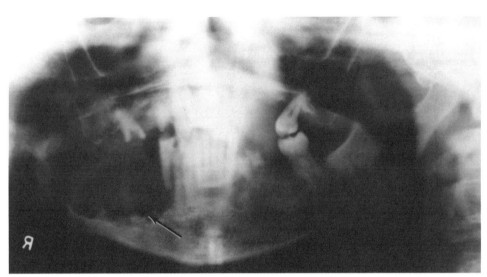

Figure 16–3
Squamous cell carcinoma producing irregular bone resorption. The lesion also involved the oral soft tissues.

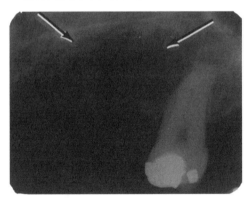

Figure 16–4
Squamous cell carcinoma of the oral mucosa invades the alveolar bone and produces diffuse destruction of bone mesial to the molar.

METASTATIC CARCINOMA

The secondary carcinoma in the jaws could have metastasized from any site in the body; the most common primary sites are breast, lung, kidney, prostate, colon, stomach and testis. Metastases to the jaws are rare and represent only 1 percent of all malignant tumors of the oral region. The mandible is more frequently affected than the maxilla and the premolar and the molar regions are most commonly involved. Usually the lesions are asymptomatic and are found on routine radiographic examination. If the mandibular nerve is involved, then the clinical signs may include pain, paresthesia or anesthesia of the lip or chin. The teeth in the region of the lesion may become loosened or exfoliated. Very often, at the time of oral examination, the patient may be unaware of the presence of the primary lesion. The radiographic appearance is similar to that of squamous cell carcinoma, that is, an ill-defined destructive radiolucent lesion which may perforate the cortical plate. Radiographic appearances often simulate periodontal disease or periapical infection.

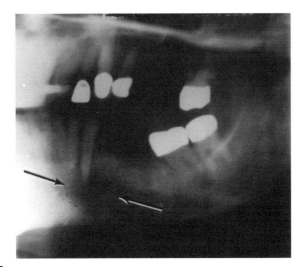

Figure 16–5
Metastatic carcinoma of the mandibular canine and premolar region in which the primary lesion was a carcinoma of the breast in a 70-year-old female.

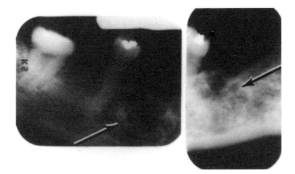

Figure 16–6
Metastatic carcinoma. Destructive radiolucency with recent history of loose teeth caused by metastatic adenocarcinoma.

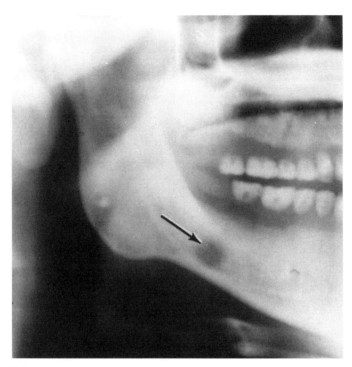

Figure 16–7
Metastatic carcinoma. Primary lesion was in the breast.

SARCOMA

Sarcomas are malignant tumors of mesodermal origin and may originate in fibrous tissue, cartilage, bone, muscle, fat or endothelial tissue. Sarcomas usually have an abundant vascular supply and, therefore, metastasize via the blood stream. Carcinomas, on the other hand, metastasize via the lymphatics. Sarcomas occur in relatively younger persons than do carcinomas. The classification of sarcomas is according to the tissues from which they are derived. The more common sarcomas are: osteosarcoma, chondrosarcoma, fibrosarcoma and Ewing's sarcoma.

OSTEOSARCOMA
(OSTEOGENIC SARCOMA)

It is a malignant tumor of bone. Although rare, osteosarcoma is the more common type of all the sarcomas. There are, in general, two types of osteosarcomas: osteoblastic (sclerosing) and osteolytic type. There are few differences in the clinical features of the two types. The osteolytic type often exhibits a rapid growth pattern and thus produces a bigger mass of bone destruction which is more susceptible to pathologic fracture.

The jaw lesion is more common in older males of mean age 33 years whereas lesions in other sites of the body occur in the younger age group of mean age 23 years. The mandible is more often involved than the maxilla. The long bones like the femur, tibia and humerus are most frequently affected. When the tumor occurs in the jaws, the chief complaint is the presence of a rapidly growing swelling and pain. The affected teeth may be loosened, displaced and paresthesia may develop. Osteosarcoma arises frequently in bones subjected to either trauma, therapeutic x-radiation or Paget's disease. Osteosarcomas are prone to develop hematogenous metastases, mainly in the lungs.

The earliest radiographic sign is a widening of the periodontal ligament space or a radiolucency around one or more teeth. Later on, the lesion assumes an osteolytic radiolucent form, an osteoblastic radiopaque form or a mixed radiolucent image with radiopaque foci. The malignant nature of the disease gives it irregular, ill-defined borders. There is expansion and destruction of the cortical plates. In one-third of the cases, thin spicules of new bone extend outwards away from the bone cortex, producing the characteristic sunray, sunburst or fan-shaped appearance.

CHONDROSARCOMA

It is a malignant tumor of cartilaginous tissue which predominantly occurs in adulthood and old age (third to fifth decade of life). Bones that arise from cartilaginous tissue are more liable to develop chondrosarcoma; therefore, a jaw lesion is rather rare. A jaw lesion has a poorer prognosis than those in other bones. In contrast to osteosarcoma, it rarely metastasizes and the extragnathic skeletal lesion has a better prognosis. Initially, the lesion occurs as a painless hard swelling of the bone which later produces extensive bone destruction. The teeth adjacent to the lesion may be resorbed, loosened, or exfoliated. Radiographic appearance of chondrosarcoma varies from moth-eaten radiolucencies that are solitary or multilocular to diffusely opaque lesions. Localized widening of the periodontal ligament space may also be observed. The borders of the lesion are poorly defined. In some cases, a sunray appearance may be seen.

FIBROSARCOMA

It is a malignant tumor of fibroblasts in which there is no deposition of osteoid or bone. Fibrosarcoma is more uncommon than osteosarcoma and chondrosarcoma. It may arise either in the jaw bones or in the soft tissues. The patient experiences pain, swelling, loosening of teeth and paresthesia. The tumor occurs in older patients (50 years) and in young children. As with osteosarcoma fibrosarcoma is occasionally associated with Paget's disease or may result from therapeutic irradiation. The radiographic appearance may simulate the radiolucent form of osteosarcoma, and have ill-defined borders. The teeth may be displaced.

EWING'S SARCOMA
(EWING'S TUMOR)

It is a malignant tumor of bone derived from mesenchymal connective tissue of the bone marrow. The lesion rarely occurs in the jaws, it is most common in the femur and tibia. It is a rapidly growing, highly invasive tumor with early and widespread metastasis. Pain and swelling are the most common manifestations. The radiographic appearance is that of an ill-defined destructive mottled radiolucent lesion which may be unilocular or multilocular. In the early stages, the mottled rarefaction may resemble an osteomyelitis. In later stages, it may stimulate the periosteum to produce thin layers of bone, resulting in an onion skin effect. Advanced cases may exhibit a sunburst appearance. The prognosis is very poor, most cases lead to death within a few years of diagnosis.

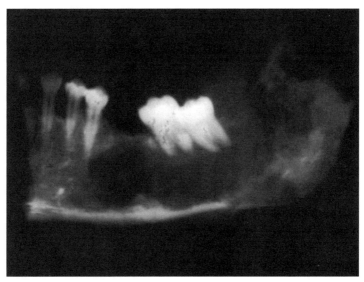

Figure 16–8
Osteosarcoma of the osteolytic type involving the mandible.

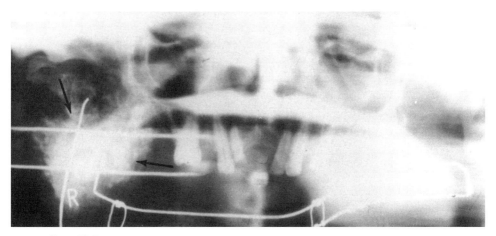

Figure 16–9
Recurrence of osteosarcoma on the right side after surgical treatment. The lesion produces the characteristic sunray appearance.

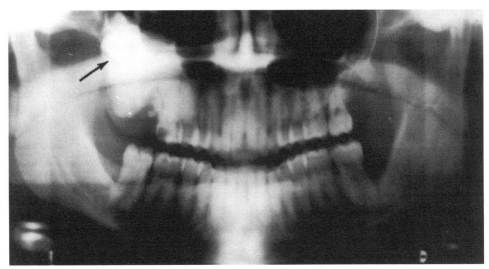

Figure 16–10
Osteosarcoma of the osteoblastic or sclerosing type in the maxilla.

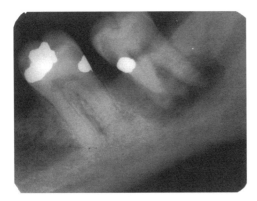

Figure 16–11
Osteosarcoma of the osteolytic type showing widening of periodontal ligament space and an apical radiolucency involving the last molar.

LEUKEMIA

Leukemia is a malignant neoplastic disease of the bone marrow and peripheral blood. The disease is characterized by overproduction of white blood cells with replacement of the normal bone marrow, circulation of abnormal cells in the blood, and infiltration of other tissues. Leukemia accounts for 5 percent of all malignancies. In children, it is the single most common cause of cancer deaths. The acute and chronic forms can occur at any age; however, the acute form generally occurs in children whereas the chronic form generally occurs in adults. Clinical manifestations include fatigability, anemia, lymphadenopathy, hepatosplenomegaly, bone and abdominal pain, secondary infection, and hemorrhagic lesions secondary to thrombocytopenia. Failure of liver and spleen is due to infiltration by malignant cells. Oral lesions include gingival bleeding, mucosal ulceration, gingival enlargement, pain and periodontitis. Radiographic findings are those of periodontal disease, severe bone loss, loss of lamina dura and loosening of teeth. Local dental cause must be ruled out to make an interpretation of leukemia.

MULTIPLE MYELOMA

Multiple myeloma is a multicentric malignant neoplasm of plasm cells in the bone marrow and affects the entire skeleton, particularly the ribs, sternum, skull, clavicles, spinal column and jaws. It occurs mainly in the older age group. Pain in the bones is the most important symptom and is accompanied by weakness, fatigue and loss of weight. The bone destruction is liable to produce pathologic fractures when the jaws are involved. Jaw pain is followed by swelling, expansion of the jaws, numbness and mobility of teeth.

The typical radiographic appearance is that of numerous small, well-defined radiolucencies, giving the characteristic punched-out appearance without a sclerotic border. Although not always present, cranial lesions are common. Sometimes there might be diffuse demineralization of various areas of the skeleton. Laboratory findings show progressive anemia, and increased serum gamma globulin which results in a reversal of the albumin/globulin ratio and increases the total serum protein level. Plasma cells are usually found in the peripheral blood and Bence Jones protein is found in the urine in at least half of the patients. Most patients suffering from multiple myeloma die within 2 to 3 years; therefore, treatment is mostly palliative.

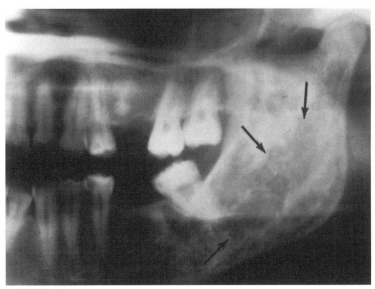

Figure 16–12
Multiple myeloma of the mandibular ramus and body showing widespread destruction of bone.

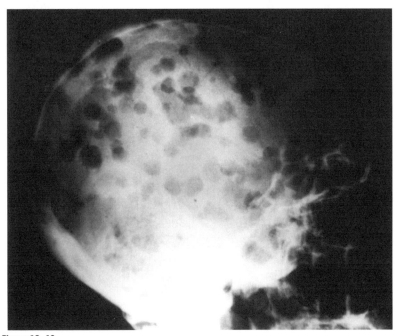

Figure 16–13
Multiple myeloma seen as multiple radiolucent lesions in skull.

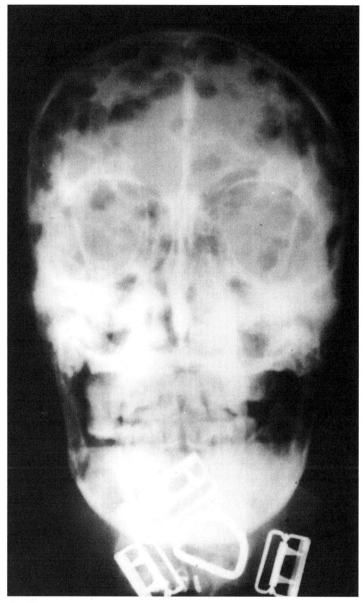

Figure 16–14
On a postero-anterior skull radiograph, multiple myeloma is seen as multiple radiolucent lesions.

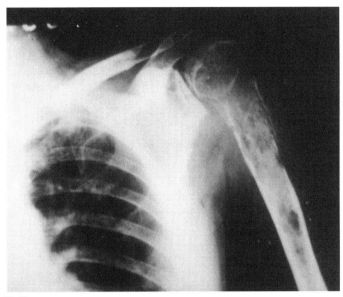

Figure 16–15
Multiple myeloma in the ribs and humerus (Courtesy Dr. A. Wuehrmann and
Dr. L. Manson-Hing).

MALIGNANT LYMPHOMAS

Malignant lymphomas are a group of immunologic neoplasms which
arise in lymphoid tissue. The various types of lymphomas are Hodgkin's
disease, lymphosarcoma, reticulum cell sarcoma and giant cell lymphoma.
Depending on the type of lymphoma, some or all of the following clinical
features may be exhibited: painless enlargement, fever, loss of weight,
anemia, generalized weakness and anorexia. All lymphomas, with the
exception of Hodgkin's disease, affect middle and older age groups. On a
radiograph, the radiolucencies are similar in appearance to periodontal
abscesses. There is loss of lamina dura around the teeth. In advanced
stages, large multilocular destructions are seen. To make a complete
diagnosis of malignant lymphoma, clinical, radiographic, microscopic and
laboratory information must be correlated.

Burkitt's Lymphoma

Burkitt's Lymphoma is a characteristic form of non-Hodgkin's lymphoma that is endemic in Africa and occurs sporadically in North America. The Epstein-Barr virus has been implicated in the etiology. Burkitt's lymphoma is primarily a tumor of childhood with occasional cases seen in young adults. Approximately 50 percent of the African cases occur in the jaws; abdominal involvement is the most common presentation for American Burkitt's lymphoma. The disease is more common in the maxilla than in the mandible. It occurs as a rapidly growing mass associated with bone destruction, loosening of teeth, and extension into adjacent soft tissues. Individuals who do not receive treatment are not likely to survive longer than 3 to 6 months. Remission occurs in 90 percent of patients who receive aggressive chemotherapy, but two-thirds of these who had advanced disease when the therapy was initiated will have relapse.

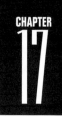

MAXILLARY
SINUS

Four pairs of paranasal sinuses surround the nasal cavities and are named from the bones in which they are located: maxillary, frontal, sphenoid, and ethmoid sinuses. The maxillary sinuses are located lateral to the nasal cavities. Each of the two sinuses is pyramidal in shape with the apex of each located near the zygomatic bone. Each maxillary sinus communicates with the nasal cavity by the ostium which opens into the middle nasal meatus under the overlapping middle nasal turbinate. Although the ostium is located at a higher level than the floor of the maxillary sinus, the normal sinus drains satisfactorily because of the action of the cilia of the pseudostratified columnar epithelium. The functions of the maxillary sinuses are: 1) to lighten the weight of the skull, 2) to give resonance to the voice, and 3) to warm and moisten the inspired air.

Most of the lesions of the maxillary sinus are clinically asymptomatic, especially those localized in the inferior portion of the antrum. These lesions do not block the free flow of fluid or gas through the ostium and thus, pressure is not increased within the sinus. Conversely, when disease conditions block the ostium, the stage is set for considerable discomfort and pain. When maxillary sinus pathoses encroach on neighboring tissues, they may produce symptoms related to the face, eye, nose and oral cavity. Pain of the maxillary bone is the most frequent symptom and may be referred to the face, eye, nose, or premolar-molar teeth. This may be accompanied by a vague headache. The facial symptoms include unilateral paresthesia, anesthesia, and feeling of fullness. Ophthalmologic symptoms include unilateral decrease in vision, pain, diplopia, epiphora and change in position of eyeball. Nasal symptoms include epistaxis, drainage, allergic rhinitis, and postnasal drip. Intraoral symptoms include pain in the premolar-molar teeth on the involved side and paresthesia or anesthesia of the gingiva and mucosa. Occasionally, a patient may complain of expansion of the alveolar process and problems with the dental occlusion. Although patients may have disturbances of the maxillary sinus, they frequently first seek professional dental service in the belief that the pain they experience is of dental origin.

Waters' projection is the most useful conventional radiographic technique to image the maxillary sinuses. In this projection, the radiographic densities of normal maxillary sinuses are the same on both sides and equal to those of the orbits. If one of the sinuses is diseased, Waters' projection will exhibit either a radiopaque (fluid) level, a sinus opacification, mucosal hyperplasia, a radiopaque growth or a loss of cortical borders of sinus. Other useful projections include periapical, panoramic, occlusal, lateral head, and Caldwell.

Variations of Normal Anatomy

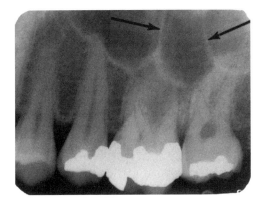

Figure 17–1
Septa in the maxillary sinus give a compartmentalized appearance to the sinus.

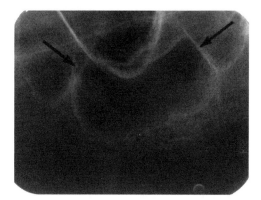

Figure 17–2

Maxillary sinus showing septa that divide it into separate compartments.

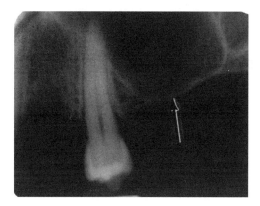

Figure 17–3

Pneumatization of the sinus. Pneumatization is the enlargement of a sinus by resorption of alveolar bone that formerly served to support a missing tooth or teeth and then occupies the edentulous space. A thin cortex remains over the alveolar ridge (arrow) to maintain a normal contour.

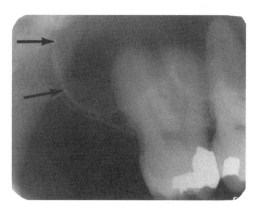

Figure 17–4

Pneumatization of the sinus. Extension of the maxillary sinus into the tuberosity as a result of pneumatization.

MAXILLARY SINUSITIS

Maxillary sinusitis (inflammation of maxillary sinus) may or may not be of dental source. The dental source of maxillary sinusitis may be periapical infection, periodontal disease, or perforation of the antral floor and antral mucosa at the time of dental extraction. Roots and foreign objects forced into the maxillary sinus at the time of operation may also be the causative factors of sinusitis. The nondental source of maxillary sinusitis may be allergic conditions, chemical irritation, or facial trauma (fracture involving a wall or walls of the maxillary sinus). The spectrum of radiographic appearances that may result from maxillary sinusitis are opacification (cloudiness) of the sinus, mucosal thickening (hyperplastic mucosa), and presence of a fluid level.

Under normal circumstances, the maxillary sinus communicates with the nasal cavity through the ostium. In sinusitis, the ostium may be blocked by a swelling of the nasal mucosa, thus causing pain and difficulty in discharging inflammatory fluid from the maxillary sinus. Maxillary sinusitis is a common complication of a nasal cold. After a few days, there is a discharge of yellowish mucopus or frank pus which may be blood-stained. The patient may complain of a sense of fullness over the cheek, especially on bending forward. Other complaints in maxillary sinusitis may include headache, facial pain and tenderness to pressure. The pain may also be referred to the premolar and molar teeth which may be sensitive or painful to percussion.

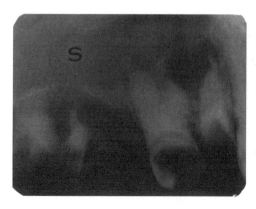

Figure 17–5
Maxillary sinusitis caused by apical infection and extensive periodontal lesions involving the molars and premolar. Notice the cloudiness (radiopacity) of the sinus (s).

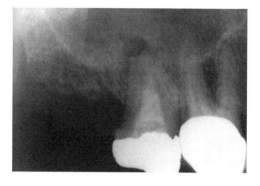

Figure 17–6

Maxillary sinusitis caused by an apical inflammatory lesion (probably, a granuloma) at the root apices of the second molar. Notice the cloudiness (radiopacity) of the sinus.

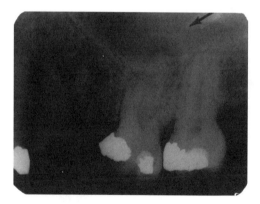

Figure 17–7

Apical infection associated with the first molar. A thickened sinus mucosa (arrow) surrounds the lesion in response to the apical infection.

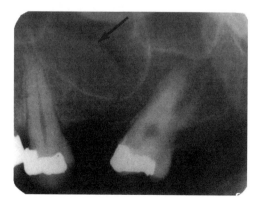

Figure 17–8

Hyperplastic mucosa. Thickened sinus mucosa (swollen mucoperiosteum). The various causes of a hyperplastic mucosa are: infection (periapical, periodontal, perforation of antral floor and mucosa), allergy, chemical irritation, foreign body and facial trauma.

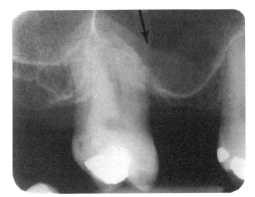

Figure 17–9
Hyperplastic mucosa.
Thickened sinus mucosa.

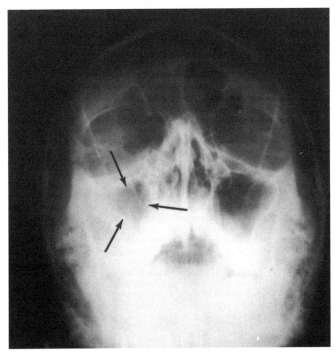

Figure 17–10
Waters' view demonstrating thickened sinus mucosa (hyperplastic mucosa) of all the walls of the right maxillary sinus. The various causes are: infection (periapical, periodontal, perforation of the antral floor and mucosa), allergy, chemical irritation, foreign body, and facial trauma.

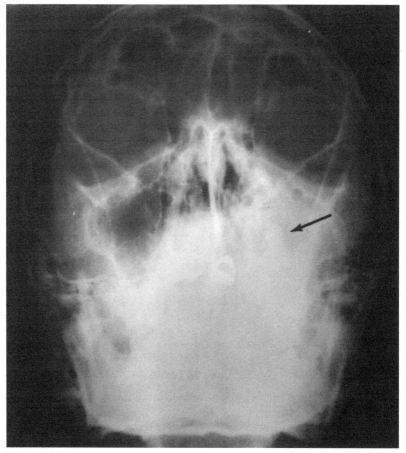

Figure 17–11

Maxillary sinusitis. Waters' view shows the radiopacity (fluid) in the involved sinus and radiolucency in the normal sinus. The unaffected sinus has the same radiolucency as the orbits. The radiopacity in the affected sinus is caused by the presence of fluid in the sinus. The most common causes of fluid in a sinus are pus caused by infection and blood resulting from trauma (fractures).

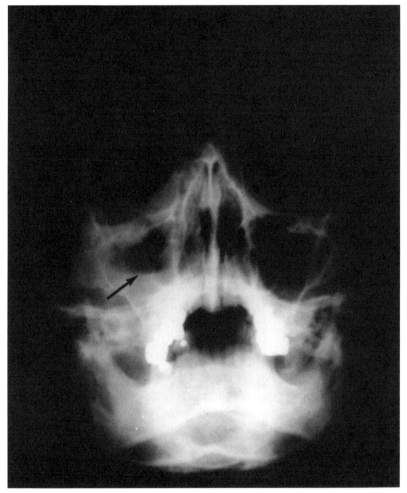

Figure 17–12
Maxillary sinusitis exhibiting a fluid level (arrow) in the right antrum.

MUCOUS RETENTION CYST

The mucous retention cyst of the antrum represents an inflammatory lesion with mucous extravasation into the submucosa of the antrum. It emanates from the antral floor as a smooth-surfaced, dome-shaped elevation. (See also Chapter 12, Cysts of the Jaws).

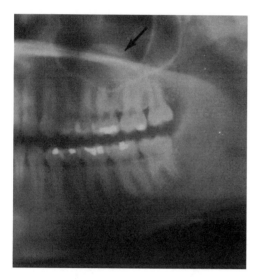

Figure 17–13

Mucous retention cyst (antral retention cyst) seen as a dome-shaped lesion on the floor of the sinus. It is usually asymptomatic but may sometimes cause some pain and tenderness in the teeth and face over the sinus. In some cases the cyst disappears spontaneously due to rupture as a result of abrupt pressure changes from sneezing or "blowing" of the nose. Later on, the cyst may reappear after a few days.

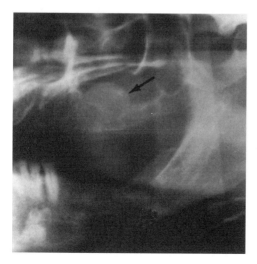

Figure 17–14

Mucous retention cyst producing a dome-shaped soft tissue radiopacity emanating from the floor of the maxillary sinus. The cyst may disappear spontaneously due to rupture and may reappear after a few days.

FOREIGN OBJECTS IN SINUS

A root of a tooth that remains after extraction may be accidentally pushed into the maxillary sinus by a clinician. The root tip acts as a nidus for calcific deposits and may form a calcified mass or stone (antrolith). A root tip in the sinus cavity does not have a surrounding lamina dura and it may change its position in the sinus with changes in head tilt. If a root tip is situated between the antral mucosa and the floor of the maxillary sinus, it does not change its position with changes in head tilt. This location of the root below the antral mucosa is not conducive for calcific deposits.

An antrolith is a stone produced by the calcification of a nidus, which may be a root tip, blood clot, mucus, or a foreign body such as a fruit pit or a gauze. An antrolith is asymptomatic and found incidentally on radiographic examination. The shapes of antroliths vary from round to very irregular.

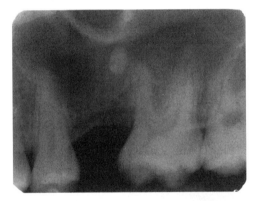

Figure 17–15

A root tip of the maxillary first molar was accidentally pushed into the sinus at the time of tooth extraction. The root tip is asymptomatic and has been present for many years. A root tip in the sinus does not have a lamina dura around it.

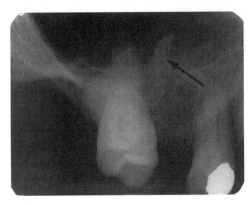

Figure 17–16

Root tip of the extracted first molar accidentally pushed into the sinus. The root tip may change its position in the sinus with changes in patient's head position. It will not change its position when it is trapped between the mucosa and the floor of the sinus.

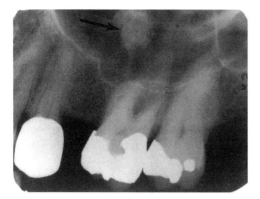

Figure 17–17

Antrolith (stone) in the maxillary sinus. Antroliths are calcified masses found in the maxillary sinus. They are formed by deposition of calcific material on a nidus such as a root fragment, bone chip, foreign object, or a mass of stagnant mucus in sites of previous inflammation.

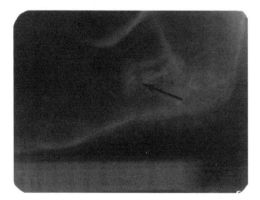

Figure 17–18

Antrolith in the maxillary sinus.

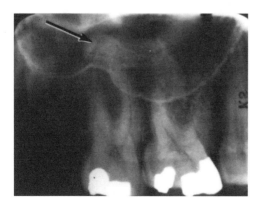

Figure 17–19

Antrolith in the maxillary sinus.

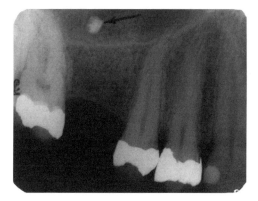

Figure 17–20
Dental cement material inadvertently pushed into the sinus during endodontic treatment of the first molar before it was extracted. The peculiar radiopacity of the dental cement distinguishes it from an antrolith.

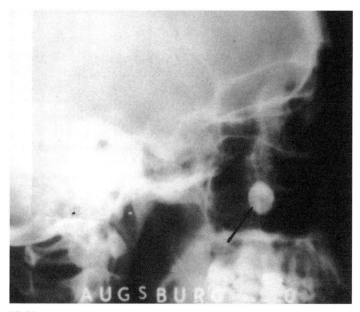

Figure 17–21
Tooth in the maxillary sinus. Sometimes a tooth in the maxillary sinus may be associated with an odontogenic cyst in the sinus. (Courtesy Dr. A. Acevedo).

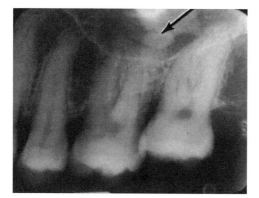

Figure 17–22
A supernumerary microdont in the maxillary sinus.

ORO-ANTRAL FISTULA

An oro-antral fistula is formed by a break in the floor of the maxillary sinus producing a communication between the maxillary sinus and the oral cavity. Thus, the oral cavity indirectly communicates with the nasal cavity via the oro-antral fistula and the ostium of the maxillary sinus. An oro-antral fistula usually arises subsequent to tooth extraction, usually in the maxillary premolar and molar regions. The clinician often becomes aware of the opening in the sinus floor during the surgical procedure. Sometimes the communication may develop a few days after the procedure. The patient frequently complains of regurgitation of food through the nose while eating and may be aware of air entering the mouth through the nose during eating and smoking. In some patients the communication between the sinus and oral cavity may remain patent and still be devoid of erythema and purulent discharge. In other patients, the inflammation in the antral cavity may discharge an exudate through the unobstructed oro-antral fistula. Sinus infection may also produce postnasal drip. In some cases the oro-antral fistula may eventually be blocked by a hyperplastic growth of the sinus mucosa or by an antral polyp herniating through the fistula.

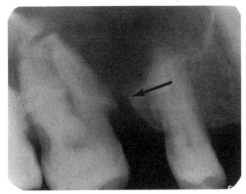

Figure 17–23

Oro-antral fistula formed by a break in the floor of the maxillary sinus between the premolar and molar. It is a pathologic tract that connects the oral cavity to the maxillary sinus. The patient complained of regurgitation of food through the nose while eating. The patient also felt air entering his mouth during eating and smoking. Sinus infection may result in postnasal drip.

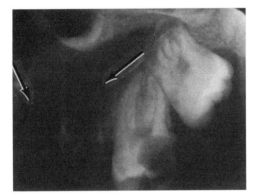

Figure 17–24

Oro-antral fistula at the site of the extracted second premolar and first molar. Patient had the usual complaint of regurgitation of food through the nose.

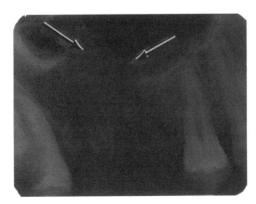

Figure 17–25

Oro-antral fistula at the site of the extracted first molar and second premolar. The mucosa of the sinus has proliferated over the fistula (arrows).

CYSTS, ODONTOGENIC AND NONODONTOGENIC

Any cyst of the maxilla, odontogenic and nonodontogenic, may slowly expand and grow into the maxillary sinus. The two most common cysts to involve the sinus are the radicular and the dentigerous cysts. A radicular cyst or a granuloma may elevate the sinus floor and produce a round shape with a thin radiopaque border, separating it from the sinus. In such cases, a radicular cyst is likely to produce an oro-antral fistula after extraction of the associated tooth. A dentigerous cyst, although fairly uncommon in the maxilla, may arise in association with a maxillary third molar tooth malposed in the maxillary sinus.

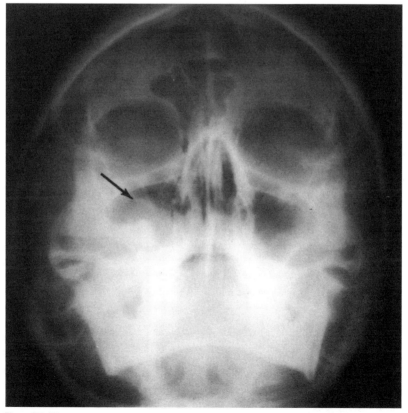

Figure 17–26
Waters' view showing a dentigerous cyst in the maxillary right sinus. A careful examination of the radiograph shows a tooth in the sinus. Any odontogenic cyst (primordial, dentigerous, radicular, or keratocyst) can encroach upon the sinus. (Courtesy Dr. A. Acevedo).

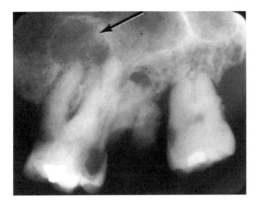

Figure 17–27
A radicular cyst at the apices of the first molar and extending into the maxillary sinus.

GENETIC, METABOLIC AND TUMOR-LIKE DISEASES

Some of the genetic, metabolic and tumor-like diseases that may commonly involve the maxillary sinus are osteopetrosis, Paget's disease, fibrous dysplasia, leontiasis ossea, and giant cell granuloma.

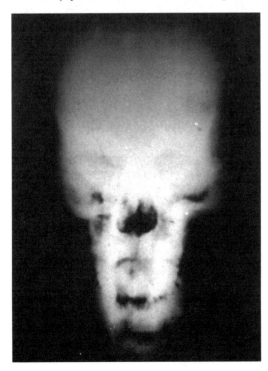

Figure 17–28
Osteopetrosis showing excessive bone accumulation in the paranasal sinuses. All the paranasal sinuses are radiopaque.

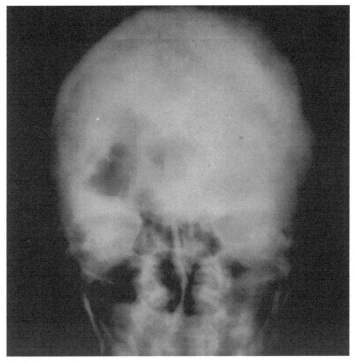

Figure 17–29

Paget's disease showing abnormal bone which usually does not penetrate but encircles the sinus. Notice the cotton-wool appearance of the skull.

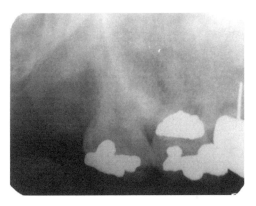

Figure 17–30

Fibrous dysplasia has encroached upon and obliterated most of the sinus cavity. The lesion has a "ground glass" appearance.

TUMORS

Some of the tumors that may commonly involve the maxillary sinus are squamous cell carcinoma, osteoma, ameloblastoma, cemento-ossifying fibroma, odontogenic myxoma, odontoma, and osteogenic sarcoma.

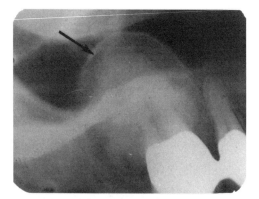

Figure 17–31

Osteoma in the floor of the maxillary sinus may be misdiagnosed for a mucous retention cyst. Notice the distinguishing presence of the trabeculae in the lesion. Osteoma is the most common of the benign nonodontogenic tumors in the paranasal sinuses.

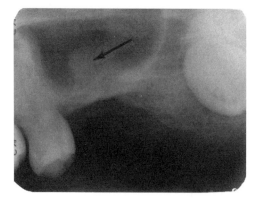

Figure 17–32

Osteoma in the floor of the maxillary sinus.

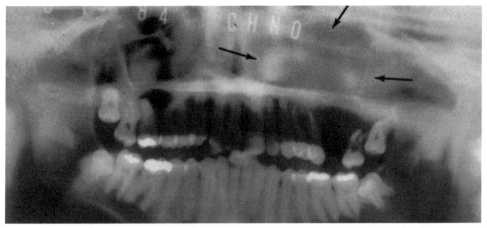

Figure 17–33

Ameloblastoma of the left maxillary sinus. The patient had pain, swelling, blurred vision and blockage of nose. Ameloblastoma is the most common benign odontogenic tumor affecting the paranasal sinuses.

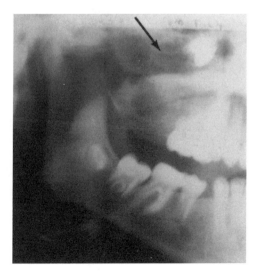

Figure 17–34

Ameloblastic fibro-odontoma in the left maxillary sinus in a 12-year-old patient. There are radiopacities in the radiolucency associated with the displaced maxillary molar.

361

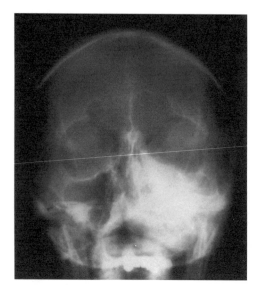

Figure 17–35

Waters' view showing a cementifying fibroma (ossifying fibroma) occluding, and producing expansion of the whole left maxillary sinus. A similar appearance may sometimes be seen in fibrous dysplasia.

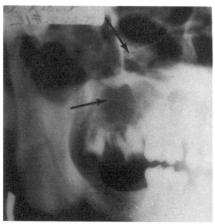

Figure 17–36

Odontogenic myxoma in the right maxillary sinus.

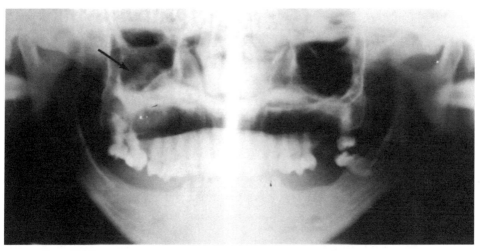

Figure 17–37

Squamous cell carcinoma in the right maxillary sinus producing destruction of the sinus floor and walls. Clinically the lesion extended into the oral soft tissues. Squamous cell carcinoma is the most common malignant tumor of the paranasal sinuses.

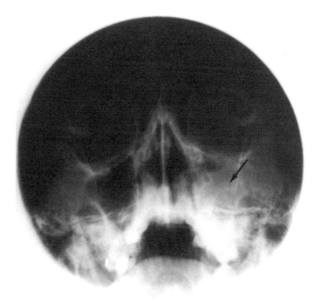

Figure 17–38

Squamous cell carcinoma of the left maxillary sinus as seen on a Waters' projection. Notice the destruction (disappearance) of the walls and floor of the sinus.

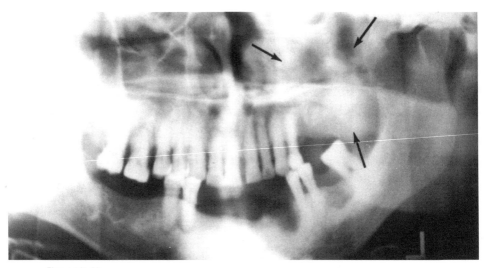

Figure 17–39

Osteosarcoma showing expansion of the left maxillary sinus. A squamous cell carcinoma could also give a similar radiographic appearance and expansion. Notice the destruction (disappearance) of the walls and floor of the sinus.

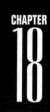

GENETIC AND METABOLIC DISEASES

I. GENETIC DISEASES

Ectodermal Dysplasia

Cherubism

Osteogenesis Imperfecta

Osteopetrosis

Cleidocranial Dysostosis

Craniofacial Dysostosis (Crouzon's Syndrome)

Mandibulofacial Dysostosis (Treacher Collins Syndrome)

Achondroplasia

Clefts of the Lip and Palate

Pierre Robin Syndrome

Sickle Cell Anemia

Thalassemia

Hemifacial Hypoplasia

Hemifacial Hypertrophy

Gardner's Syndrome

II. METABOLIC DISEASES

Paget's Disease

Hyperparathyroidism

Hypoparathyroidism

Hyperpituitarism

Hypopituitarism

Hyperthyroidism

Hypothyroidism

Diabetes Mellitus

Cushing's Syndrome

Rickets and Osteomalacia

Hypophosphatasia

Osteoporosis

Scleroderma

Infantile Cortical Hyperostosis

ECTODERMAL DYSPLASIA

Ectodermal dysplasia is a syndrome which is transmitted as an X-linked recessive disorder and occurs almost exclusively in males. This hereditary developmental disturbance affects the ectodermal tissues like hair, fingernails, sweat glands and teeth. Patients exhibit soft, smooth, thin, dry skin with partial or complete absence of sweat glands. Since these patients cannot perspire normally because of the agenesis of sweat glands, they are unable to endure warm temperatures. The hair of the scalp and those of the eyebrows tend to be fine, scanty, blonde and resemble lanugo. Body hair is sparse or absent. The finger and toe nails are small and deformed or absent. The bridge of the nose may be depressed and the supraorbital ridges may be very prominent (frontal bossing). Oral manifestations include total anodontia or hypodontia. The teeth which are present are often malformed; frequently they are cone-shaped.

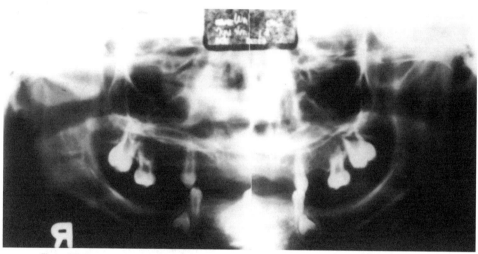

Figure 18–1
Ectodermal dysplasia. Patient exhibiting hypodontia.

CHERUBISM
(HEREDITARY FIBROUS DYSPLASIA OF THE JAWS, FAMILIAL INTRAOSSEOUS SWELLINGS OF THE JAWS, FAMILIAL MULTILOCULAR CYSTIC DISEASE OF THE JAWS)

Cherubism is a hereditary condition that produces firm, painless swellings that occur bilaterally in the jaws, especially over the mandibular angles. This autosomal dominant disease is usually detected between the ages of 2 and 7 years. The mandible is more frequently affected and produces a full, round lower face similar to those of cherubs portrayed in Renaissance religious paintings. Often the eyes are upturned to reveal the white sclera beneath. In some cases, where the maxilla is involved, the skin of the cheeks appears to be stretched. This benign fibro-osseous disease does not affect the other bones of the body. The bony defects contain soft tissue that is histologically similar, if not identical, to a giant cell granuloma.

On a radiograph of the mandible, the expansion of the buccal and lingual cortical plates is seen on occlusal and postero-anterior views. The mandibular body and rami are frequently involved. Enlargement of the maxilla is at the expense of the maxillary sinuses. The lesion consists of multiple cyst-like radiolucencies which are located bilaterally in the jaws. These bilateral multilocular radiolucencies are a characteristic feature of cherubism. The teeth may be unerupted and displaced. Some of the teeth appear to be floating in the cyst-like spaces. This benign, self-limited disorder tends to regress after puberty, thus eliminating the need for surgical intervention. Treatment, if necessary, consists of recontouring the bone for cosmetic reasons after the lesions have stabilized in size.

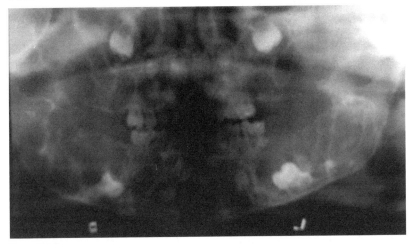

Figure 18–2
Cherubism. Panoramic radiograph showing extensive multilocular radiolucent lesions of the mandible and maxilla.

OSTEOGENESIS IMPERFECTA (BRITTLE BONES DISEASE, FRAGILITAS OSSIUM, LOBSTEIN'S DISEASE)

Osteogenesis imperfecta is a hereditary disorder of connective tissues; that is, there is an inborn error of collagen metabolism which produces an abnormality in the organic matrix of bone. Some cases occur as autosomal dominant traits whereas others occur as spontaneous mutations (idiopathic). The development of bones is poor and, therefore, results in their fragility, porosity and proneness to fracture. Although the fractures heal, the new bone formation is of imperfect quality. An exuberance of callus may be formed at the sites of repeated fractures. Bowing of the limbs and angulation deformities occur at previous fracture sites. A characteristic clinical feature is that of a patient having pale blue sclera caused by the pigmented choroid coat showing through the thinned sclera. Early hearing loss in a patient or a member of a family with a history of fragile bones is highly suggestive of the disorder.

The oral findings are similar to those seen in dentinogenesis imperfecta in which the crowns of teeth are of opalescent hue. Like bone, the dentin is poorly calcified and, therefore, the crowns fracture easily. The exposed dentin undergoes rapid attrition. Radiographic appearance is that of teeth constricted near their cervical portions and having thin, short roots. The pulp chambers and canals are calcified and obliterated. There are types I, II, III and IV of osteogenesis imperfecta, each having specific clinical features. It is the most common inherited bone disease and owing to its variable clinical expression, many mildly affected patients remain undiagnosed.

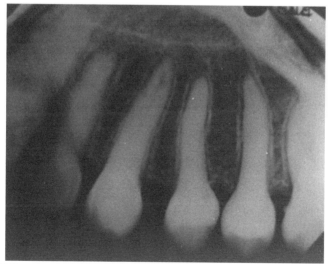

Figure 18–3

Osteogenesis imperfecta. The dental changes are similar to those of dentinogenesis imperfecta: teeth constricted near the cervical portions, thin and short roots, calcification of pulp chambers and root canals. Clinically, the crowns are of opalescent hue.

OSTEOPETROSIS
(ALBERS-SCHÖNBERG DISEASE,
MARBLE BONE DISEASE)

Osteopetrosis, also known as Albers-Schönberg disease or marble bone disease, is a rare disease of unknown etiology. In most cases heredity seems to play a role. The infantile type (malignant form) is inherited as an autosomal recessive trait whereas the adult type (benign form) is inherited as an autosomal dominant trait. Although both forms are congenital in origin, the adult type may not be noticed until later in childhood or adulthood. Osteopetrosis is characterized by skeletal, hematologic, and neurologic abnormalities. In skeletal abnormalities, there is an increased calcification and thickening of cortical and spongy portions of the entire skeletal (osseous) system. The formation of bone is normal but the resorption of bone is reduced owing to a reduction in osteoclastic activity. The bones become fragile and susceptible to fracture. In osteopetrosis, multiple fractures result from excessive mineralization; whereas in osteogenesis imperfecta, the fractures result from bone resorption. In hematologic abnormalities, secondary anemia occurs due to a reduction of available marrow because of extensive deposition of dense bone in the bone marrow. There may be enlargement of spleen and liver (hepatosplenomegaly). In neurologic abnormalities the excess bone formation narrows the various foramina in the base of the skull; this may produce blindness, deafness, diabetes insipidus, facial palsy, and neuralgic pain, depending on the nerve being compressed. The relative avascularity of the bone makes it vulnerable to infection, especially at the time of tooth extraction and results in osteomyelitis. Another complication that may result at the time of extraction is that the bone may fracture easily. In the infantile type of osteopetrosis, most patients die before age 20 as a result of anemia or infection.

In the clinically benign adult form, the life expectancy is usually normal; the disease may not be diagnosed until the third or fourth decade. Osteopetrosis can be diagnosed solely on the basis of appropriate radiographic findings. The bones of the body show greatly increased density; their medullary cavities are replaced by bone. A lateral skull radiograph shows an increased radiopacity due to increased thickness of the bones in the skull, calvarium and all the structures at the base. Dental defects include delayed eruption, early loss of teeth, missing teeth, malformed roots and crowns.

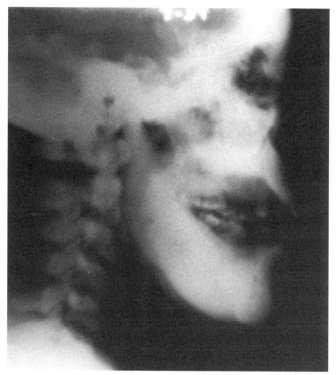

Figure 18–4
Osteopetrosis. Lateral skull radiograph shows dense calcification of jaws and skull resulting in loss of trabeculae. All the sinuses are obliterated with bone.

CLEIDOCRANIAL DYSOSTOSIS

Cleidocranial dysostosis is an inherited skeletal anomaly which affects primarily the skull, clavicle and dentition. Some of the cases occur spontaneously but most are inherited in an autosomal dominant mode. The skull findings are brachycephaly (reduced anteroposterior dimension but increased skull width), delayed or failed closure of the fontanelles, and the presence of open skull sutures and multiple wormian bones. There is pronounced frontal, parietal and occipital bossing. Underdeveloped maxilla and paranasal sinuses result in maxillary micrognathia. The mandible is not involved; however, the maxillary hypoplasia gives the mandible a relative prognathic appearance. The syndrome is notable for aplasia or hypoplasia of the clavicles. Some patients have hypermobility of shoulders and can bring them forward until they meet in the midline. The neck appears long and narrow, and the shoulders markedly drooped. Oral manifestations exhibit a high narrow arched palate. Often there may be a true or submucosal cleft palate. Crowding of teeth is produced by retention of deciduous teeth, delayed eruption of permanent teeth, and the presence of a large number of unerupted supernumerary teeth. The supernumerary teeth are mainly found in the premolar and molar regions. The affected individuals do not need any treatment for the syndrome and often enjoy normal life.

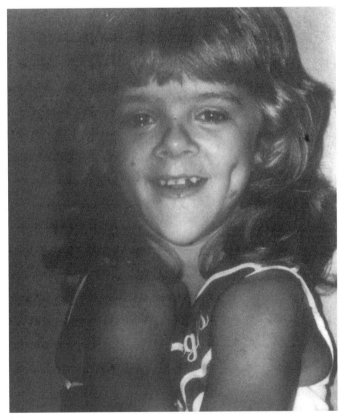

Figure 18–5

Cleidocranial dysostosis. In the absence of clavicles, the patient can bring the shoulders forward towards the midline. Note the underdeveloped maxilla.

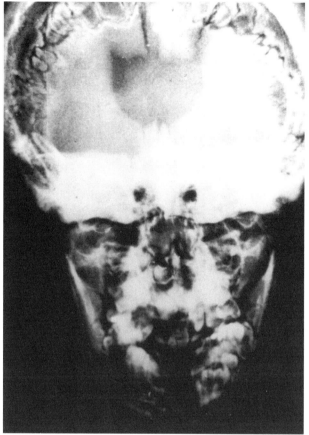

Figure 18–6

Cleidocranial dysostosis. Postero-anterior skull radiograph shows delayed closure of sutures and fontanelles, and presence of multiple wormian bones. Multiple supernumerary teeth are present.

CRANIOFACIAL DYSOSTOSIS (CROUZON'S DISEASE)

Craniofacial dysostosis, also known as Crouzon's disease, is an inherited anomaly characterized by a variety of cranial deformities. In this autosomal dominant disorder, the skull reveals early closure of all cranial sutures. Premature closure of these sutures (craniosynostosis) can initiate changes in the brain secondary to increased intracranial pressure. The resulting increased intracranial pressure produces malformation of the skull, including frontal bossing. Facial malformation consists of hypoplasia of the maxilla with a relative mandibular prognathism and a high arched palate. The maxillary hypoplasia produces the characteristic facies often described as frog-like. The eyes are set wide apart (hypertelorism) and protrude (exophthalmos) with divergent strabismus. The deformities of the cranial bones and orbital cavities are the result of the fusion of sutures and increased intracranial pressure. The life expectancy for the patients is, in general, normal. Many have progressive visual impairment and a few may have mental retardation. Surgical intervention may be necessary to relieve intracranial pressure. Radiographic examination of the skull reveals the absence of cranial sutures and the presence of multiple radiolucent cranial markings (digital impressions) covering the inner surface of the cranial vault.

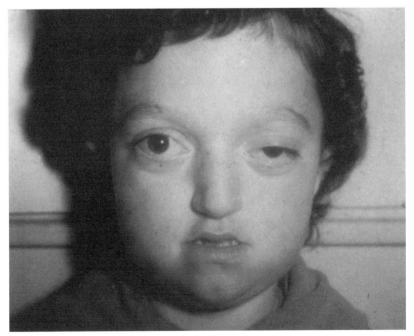

Figure 18–7
Cruzon's disease (craniofacial dysostosis). Facial malformation shows hypoplasia of maxilla with mandibular prognathism. Eyes exhibit hypertelorism, exophthalmos and divergent strabismus. (Courtesy Dr. William Ledoux).

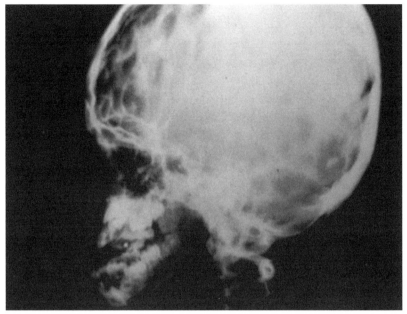

Figure 18–8

Cruzon's disease (craniofacial dysostosis). Lateral skull radiograph shows early closure of all cranial sutures. Note the prominent digital markings. (Courtesy Dr. William Ledoux).

MANDIBULOFACIAL DYSOSTOSIS (TREACHER COLLINS SYNDROME)

Mandibulofacial dysostosis, also known as Treacher Collins syndrome, is a rare hereditary developmental anomaly which is transmitted by an autosomal dominant mode of inheritance; some are spontaneous mutations. In the fully expressed syndrome, the facial appearance is characteristic and is often described as bird-like or fish-like. The syndrome is characterized by hypoplasia of the facial bones, particularly the zygomatic bone and the mandible. The underdeveloped zygomaticomaxillary complex leads to a clinically severe midface deficiency. The external ears are malformed (deformed pinnas) and sometimes the middle and inner ears are also affected, resulting in partial or complete deafness. A striking feature is the antimongoloid obliquity or downward slanting of the palpebral fissures and notched or linear colobomas of the outer third of the lower eyelids. Macrostomia may be present. The palate is usually high and sometimes clefted. Dental malocclusions are very common. On radiographic examination, the zygomatic bone (cheek) often appears to be underdeveloped or completely absent. There is also underdevelopment of the paranasal sinuses. The mastoid bone is often sclerotic; that is, the mastoid air cells are absent or reduced. The life expectancy of these patients is normal. Some patients may need ear surgery and hearing aids.

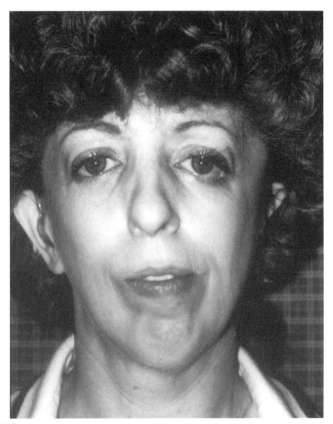

Figure 18–9

Treacher Collins syndrome (mandibulofacial dysostosis). Note the characteristic facial appearance: downward slanting of palpebral fissures, colobomas of outer third of lower eyelids, depressed cheek bones, receding chin, and a nose that appears relatively large.

ACHONDROPLASIA

Achondroplasia is a hereditary condition (autosomal dominant) producing disturbance in the formation and development of bones ossified in cartilage; that is, the normal process of cartilaginous bone growth is retarded and ceases prematurely. As a result, the bones derived from cartilage are short but of normal width. Ossification of bones derived from membrane (intramembranous ossification) proceeds normally. Thus, the skull vault (derived from membrane) seems large in proportion to the base (derived from cartilage) and the vertebral column long in proportion to the limbs. The lack of growth at the epiphyses of long bones produces extremities which are short in comparison with the torso. An achondroplastic dwarf is quite short, with short muscular extremities, brachycephalic skull and bowed legs. The elbows cannot often be straightened because the joints exhibit limitation of motion. They are endowed with normal intelligence, unusual strength and agility. Radiographs of the skull show that the maxilla is retruded because of the restriction of growth of the base of the skull. The retrusion produces a relative mandibular prognathism. The disparity in size of the two jaws produces obvious malocclusion and a saddle-nose profile. The dentition is usually normal, but may show congenitally missing teeth and disturbance in the shape of those present. Achondroplastic dwarfism must not be mistaken with pituitary dwarfism; in the latter, the size of the limbs is in proportion to the size of the body.

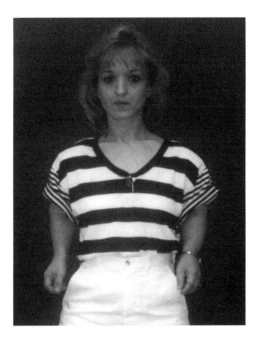

Figure 18–10
Achondroplasia. Patient shows extremities which are short in comparison with the torso. Achondroplastic dwarfism must not be mistaken with pituitary dwarfism; in the latter, the size of the limbs is in proportion to the size of the torso.

CLEFTS OF THE JAW BONES

Clefts of the jaw bones result from complete or partial failure of the developmental processes to fuse during embryonic life. The Japanese have a higher frequency of cleft palate than do whites and the incidence is lowest in American blacks. The incidence of cleft lip or cleft palate is about 1 in 800 infants that are born. Clefts of the jaws cause severe functional problems of speech, mastication, and deglutition. Cleft lip causes difficulty with suckling whereas cleft palate causes problems with regurgitation of food and liquid into the nose as well as problems with speech. Clefts can involve the lip, hard palate, soft palate, uvula, alveolar process or all of them. When the alveolar ridge is involved, it is usually in the region of the maxillary lateral incisor. Clefts may be unilateral or bilateral. A combination of cleft lip and palate is the most common of the various clefts. Cleft lip generally occurs at about the sixth to seventh week in utero whereas cleft palate occurs at about the eighth week in embryonic development. Isolated cleft lip is more common and more severe in males whereas isolated cleft palate is more common in females. The occurrence of mandibular lip or jaw clefts are extremely rare.

Radiographs are useful in determining the exact site of the cleft, the amount of bone present, and the position of the teeth near the cleft. Both the dentitions, deciduous and permanent, may be affected. Supernumerary, missing and malpositioned teeth are often associated with clefts. Cleft lips are usually repaired surgically at about one month of age. Cleft palates are usually repaired after 18 months of age; that is, after speech patterns are well-established and it is developmentally late enough for the growth centers to be disturbed.

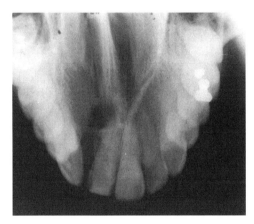

Figure 18–11
Cleft of the maxilla situated between the maxillary lateral incisor and canine.

PIERRE ROBIN SYNDROME

In Pierre Robin syndrome, mandibular retrognathia and hypoplasia is the primary malformation. Along with the severe micrognathia, the other clinical presentations include cleft palate and glossoptosis (posteriorly placed tongue which falls back into the airway). Respiratory and feeding problems are prevalent and may result in episodic airway obstruction, with infant hypoxia and malnutrition. The associated respiratory difficulty, if not recognized, may result in death.

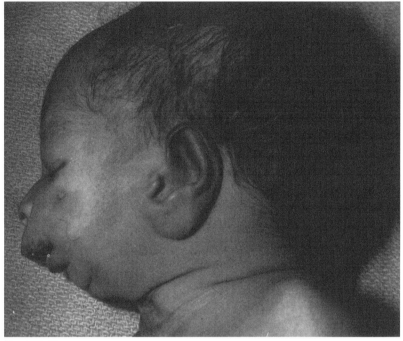

Figure 18–12
Pierre Robin syndrome. Infant exhibiting severe micrognathia of the mandible. (Courtesy Dr. Jim Weir).

SICKLE CELL ANEMIA

Sickle cell anemia is an inherited disorder which occurs almost exclusively in black individuals. It is a chronic hemolytic anemia characterized by abnormal hemoglobin, which under low oxygen tension results in sickling of the red blood cells. Thus, the red blood cells have a reduced capacity to carry oxygen to the tissues. They also adhere to the vascular endothelium and clog the capillaries. During a mild attack, the patient complains of weakness, easy fatigability, shortness of breath, muscle and joint pain. Patients may exhibit general signs of anemia and jaundice. During the crisis state there is severe abdominal, muscle and joint pain, high temperature; circulatory collapse may result. The disease occurs in children and adolescents. Many patients die of complications before the age of 40 years, although some may have a normal life span. Radiographic appearance is principally caused by hyperplasia of bone marrow of several bones in the body. The skull demonstrates a widening of the diploic spaces and thinning of the inner and outer tables of bone. In some cases there may be a loss of the outer table of bone which may give rise to a hair-on-end appearance. Osteoporosis may be observed in the mandible with coarse mandibular trabeculae giving a stepladder appearance.

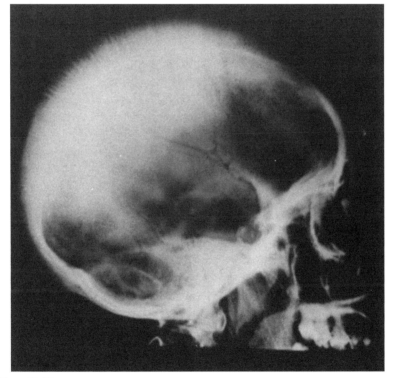

Figure 18–13
Sickle cell anemia. Lateral skull radiograph shows thicker than normal cranial vault and linear markings of hair-on-end appearance.

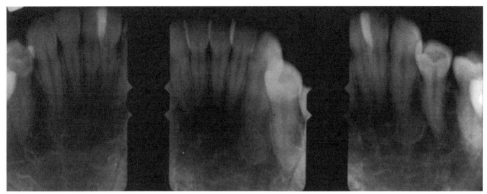

Figure 18–14

Sickle cell anemia. Enlarged marrow spaces with the trabeculae giving a stepladder appearance.

THALASSEMIA
(COOLEY'S ANEMIA, MEDITERRANEAN ANEMIA, ERYTHROBLASTIC ANEMIA)

Thalassemia, also called Cooley's anemia, is a hereditary chronic anemia which results from abnormal red blood cells having difficulties in hemoglobin synthesis. The red blood cells thus have a reduced hemoglobin content and a shortened life span. Thalassemia was once more prevalent in people living in or originating from the lands around the Mediterranean Sea. This disease is now widely distributed. Radiographic examination shows the expansion of the bone marrow spaces with generalized osteoporosis. The skull exhibits a wide diploe. Sometimes the loss of the outer table of bone may give rise to the characteristic hair-on-end appearance of the skull.

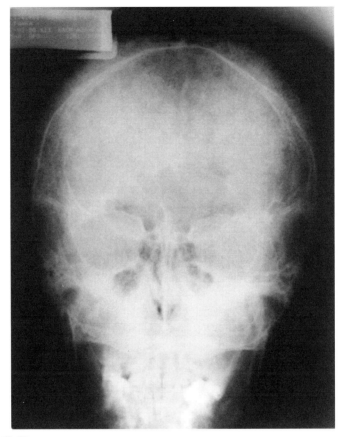

Figure 18–15

Thalassemia. Postero-anterior skull radiograph shows the characteristic hair-on end appearance. (Courtesy Drs. Jan Hes, Isaäc van derWaal and Kommer de Man).

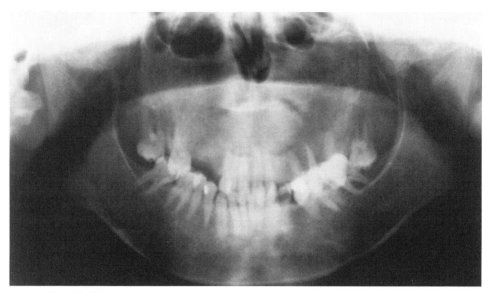

Figure 18–16

Thalassemia. Panoramic radiograph shows generalized rarefaction, thinning of cortical bone, and enlarged marrow spaces with thin trabeculation. (Courtesy Drs. Jan Hes, et al.)

HEMIFACIAL HYPOPLASIA

Hemifacial hypoplasia may have its onset at birth or at any time up to the cessation of facial growth. There is progressive failure of growth of the affected side with the result that there is a reduced dimension of the involved side of the face. There may be malocclusion on the affected side but the teeth are of normal size and shape. Radiographic examination reveals a reduction in the size of the bones on the affected side, especially the condyle, coronoid process and the overall dimension of the body and ramus of the mandible.

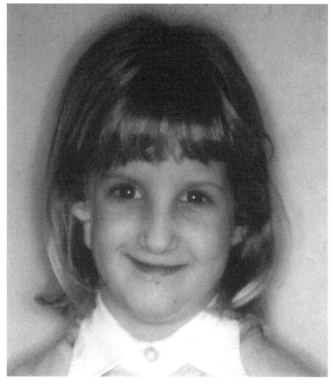

Figure 18–17
 Hemifacial hypoplasia. The affected side of the face is smaller than the normal side. Note the crumpled and distorted pinna of the external ear on the involved side. (Courtesy Dr. William Ledoux).

HEMIFACIAL HYPERTROPHY

Hemifacial hypertrophy begins during youth, sometimes at birth, and usually continues throughout the growing years. It may be characterized by gross body asymmetry or may involve only a specific region of the body. There is progressive growth of half of the face and jaws to unusual proportions. The condition is often associated with other abnormalities including mental deficiency, skin abnormalities (excessive secretions by sebaceous and sweat glands) and compensatory scoliosis. Craniofacial findings include asymmetry of the frontal bone, maxilla, palate, mandible, alveolar process, condyles and associated soft tissue. The pinna of the ear is often remarkably enlarged. Dental malocclusion is common owing to asymmetric growth of the maxilla, mandible, and alveolar process. Radiographic examination of the skulls of these patients reveals enlargement of the bones on the affected side.

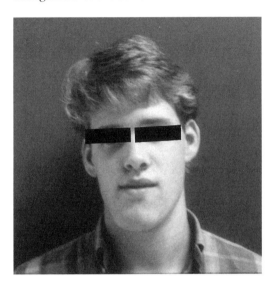

Figure 18–18
Hemifacial hypertrophy. Facial asymmetry resulting from progressive growth of half of the face.

GARDNER'S SYNDROME

Gardner's syndrome is an inherited autosomal dominant disorder. This syndrome complex is characterized by skeletal, gastrointestinal, dermatologic and dental manifestations. The skeletal manifestations include multiple osteomas, especially of the skull and jaws. The gastrointestinal manifestations include multiple intestinal polyps of the colon and rectum but rarely involve the small intestine. The dermatologic manifestations include multiple epidermal cysts and fibromas of the skin. The dental manifestations include multiple impacted supernumerary teeth, failure of permanent teeth to erupt and tendency to form odontomas. Patients afflicted with Gardner's syndrome should be diagnosed and treated in the early stages otherwise, they will develop and then die of colonic carcinoma.

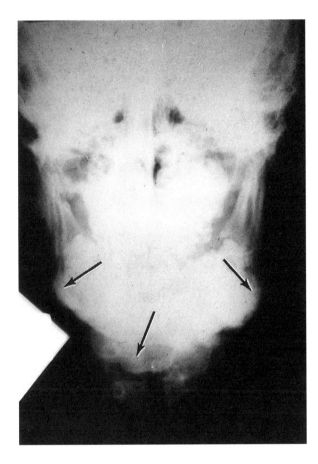

Figure 18–19
Gardner's syndrome. Postero-anterior skull radiograph shows multiple osteomas (arrows). (Courtesy Dr. Jim Cade).

PAGET'S DISEASE
(OSTEITIS DEFORMANS)

Paget's disease, also called osteitis deformans, is a disease of unknown etiology. The incidence increases in older individuals, especially those over the age of 40 years. Pain in a bone may be mistaken for arthritis. The initial lesion is one of destruction by resorption; later an excessive amount of bone is deposited in a haphazard fashion with a diminution of vascularity of the lesion. The new bone is of poor quality and may result in increased bone fragility and a tendency to fracture. In fact, pathologic fracture is one of the most common complications of Paget's disease. The neurologic

387

symptoms in Paget's disease develop gradually and consist of bone pain, severe headache, deafness, loss of sight, dizziness, facial paralysis, mental disturbance and weakness. The disease may be monostotic or polyostotic. When polyostotic, the bones most prominently affected are those of the axial skeleton which include the skull, vertebral column, extremities and maxilla. There is progressive enlargement of the skull, bowing deformity of long bones and dorsal kyphosis (spinal curvature). The patient develops a waddling gait. The jaws are involved in only 20 percent of cases; the maxilla is more frequently affected than the mandible (3:1 ratio). In some instances, both jaws are involved. Ultimately the alveolar ridge widens with a relative flattening of the palatal vault. The enlargement of the maxilla and/or the mandible results in migration, spacing of the teeth and malocclusion. Dentures may have to be remade periodically to accommodate the increase in jaw size. An important diagnostic feature of Paget's disease is that the serum alkaline phosphatase level is increased to extreme limits although serum calcium and phosphate levels are normal. The disease often proceeds with exacerbations and remissions. During remissions the level of alkaline phosphatase is usually normal.

On a radiograph, in the early stages, the density of bone is decreased. As the disease progresses, osteoblastic activity is more than osteoclastic activity; so that apposition exceeds resorption of bone. The osteoblastic areas appear as patchy radiopacities and give the characteristic cotton-wool appearance similar to that of florid osseous dysplasia (chronic diffuse sclerosing osteomyelitis). The lamina dura around the teeth in the involved regions may be absent. The teeth may be hypercementosed only after the bony changes in the jaw are manifested. The most serious complication of Paget's disease is osteogenic sarcoma and occurs in 10 percent of the patients. On extraction of teeth in an affected part of bone, the wound healing is disturbed and may result in suppurative osteomyelitis. There is no specific treatment for Paget's disease.

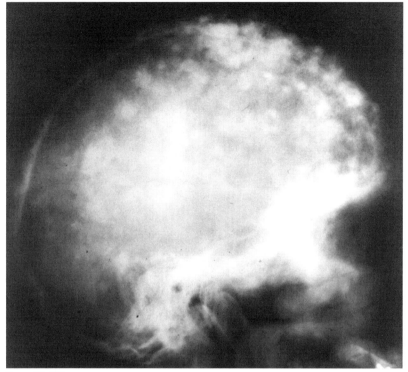

Figure 18–20A
Paget's disease. Lateral skull radiograph shows patchy radiopacities giving the characteristic cotton-wool appearance.

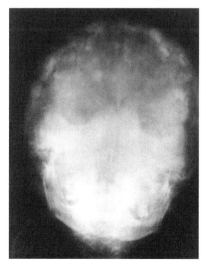

Figure 18–20B
Paget's disease showing a "cotton-wool" appearance on a postero-anterior projection of the skull.

389

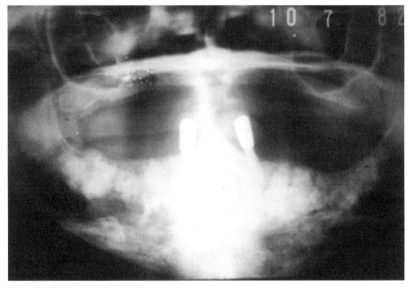

Figure 18–21

Paget's disease. Panoramic radiograph shows multiple radiopaque masses producing the characteristic cotton-wool appearance similar to that of florid osseous dysplasia.

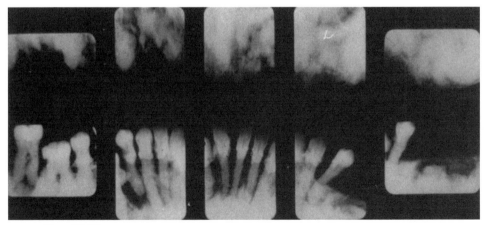

Figure 18–22

Paget's disease. Periapical radiographs show patchy radipacities of the jaws, spacing of teeth, loss of lamina dura and some hypercementosed teeth.

HYPERPARATHYROIDISM

Hyperparathyroidism is an endocrine abnormality in which there is an excess of circulating parathyroid hormone (PTH). The PTH mobilizes calcium from the skeleton and decreases renal tubular reabsorption of phosphate. Primary hyperparathyroidism is caused by a benign tumor or hyperplasia of the parathyroid gland, producing an excess quantity of PTH hormone. In primary hyperparathyroidism, the serum calcium is elevated beyond its normal 9-11 mg% range by resorption of calcium from bones and decreased renal excretion of calcium. The serum phosphorus level is decreased. Secondary hyperparathyroidism is the result of certain types of kidney diseases that cause hypocalcemia, thereby stimulating the parathyroid glands to secrete excess PTH in an attempt to elevate the serum calcium level. The serum calcium is normal to decreased and serum phosphorus is increased.

Hyperparathyroidism is a common cause of generalized rarefaction of the jaws. The skeleton undergoes generalized osteoporosis and is seen on a radiograph as having a ground glass appearance with loss of trabecular bone pattern. In a small percentage of patients there is loss of lamina dura around all the teeth. The lost lamina dura returns after successful treatment of the disorder. Late in the disease, a small number of cases develop central giant cell lesions known as brown tumors. These brown tumors appear radiographically as ill-defined radiolucencies. There is a tendency for the patients to develop renal stones. The serum alkaline phosphatase level is elevated. Increase in serum alkaline phosphatase level occurs in systemic and bone diseases whenever there is significant bone resorption or turnover.

(Note: Brown tumors are histologically identical with the central giant cell granuloma of the jaws. For this reason, hyperparathyroidism should always be ruled out in a patient with a giant cell lesion of the jaws).

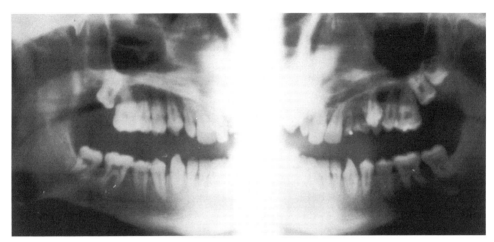

Figure 18–23
Hyperparathyroidism. Panoramic radiograph shows generalized disappearance of lamina dura and reduction in radiographic bone density in both jaws.

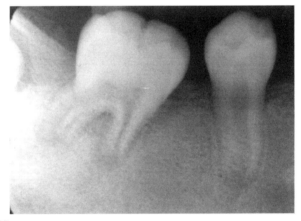

Figure 18–24
Hyperparathyroidism. Osteoporosis of bone is seen on the radiograph as having a ground glass appearance with loss of trabecular bone pattern. Also, there is loss of lamina dura.

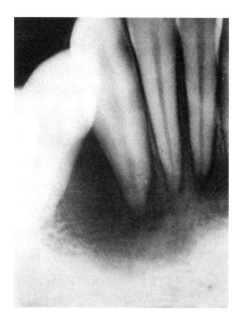

Figure 18–25
Hyperparathyroidism. Central giant cell lesions known as "brown tumors" produce ill-defined radiolucencies and disappearance of lamina dura.

HYPOPARATHYROIDISM

Hypoparathyroidism is a relatively rare disease caused by an accidental (or purposeful) removal of the parathyroid glands during surgery. The clinical syndrome is characterized by a reduction in the secretion of the parathyroid hormone. There is decreased renal tubular reabsorption of calcium and increased renal tubular reabsorption of phosphate. The resulting hypocalcemia leads to increased neuromuscular excitability with tetany. Tetany is manifested in the form of carpopedal spasm. When hypoparathyroidism occurs in children, it may cause hypoplasia of enamel and dentin, underdevelopment of the roots of forming teeth and delayed eruption. If not treated, hypoparathyroidism may cause laryngospasm and death.

HYPERPITUITARISM

In hyperpituitarism there is increased production of growth hormone, causing an overgrowth of all tissues in the body which are still capable of growth. If hyperpituitarism occurs in childhood, the result is gigantism; if it occurs in adulthood, it results in acromegaly.

In gigantism, there is relatively uniform overgrowth of soft tissues and bone, producing a fairly well-proportioned but abnormally large individual with heights of 7 feet or more. Sexual maturity is at a young age; however, impotency occurs at an early age. Radiographic examination reveals normal size teeth which are widely spaced because of increased jaw size. The posterior teeth may be hypercementosed due to functional and structural demands. The trabecular pattern is normal. A lateral view radiograph of the skull shows an enlarged cranium, an enlarged sella turcica, a prominent frontal sinus and a prognathic mandible.

In acromegaly (hyperpituitarism of adult onset), there is no further increase in height because the adult bones are incapable of increased growth because the epiphyses of bones are fused with their shafts. The sutures of the craniofacial bones are fused. However, there is subperiosteal deposition of bone, resulting in increased thickness of arms and legs. The main feature is the enlargement of the mandible, producing a Class III skeletal malocclusion. An increase in dental arch length does not occur (as in gigantism); however, anterior teeth may be spaced because of the pressure effects of macroglossia. The teeth are of normal size. The posterior teeth may be hypercementosed due to functional and structural demands. The trabecular pattern is normal. The nose, lips, tongue, and soft tissues of the hands and feet overgrow, sometimes to an abnormally large size. A lateral view radiograph demonstrates an enlarged mandible with a prognathic bite, enlarged sella turcica, frontal sinus and occipital prominence.

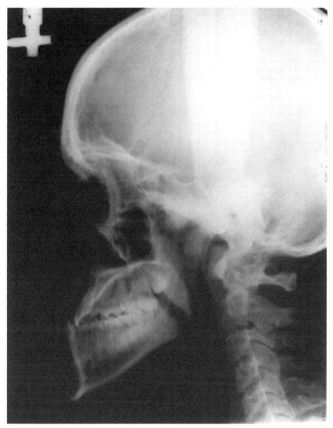

Figure 18–26

Hyperpituitarism producing acromegaly. The main feature is the enlargement of the mandible, producing a Class III skeletal malocclusion.

HYPOPITUITARISM

In hypopituitarism there is reduced secretion of pituitary hormones. It results in a condition called pituitary dwarfism in which the person is of small stature and proportionate in body. Mental development is normal. Jaw growth is retarded, resulting in a small vertical dimension and a small arch length. The teeth are of normal size. Crowding of teeth and malocclusion results because of disproportion in the sizes of the jaws and teeth. Radiographs of extremities show marked retardation of osseous development. Periapical radiographs show retention of deciduous teeth, delayed eruption of permanent teeth and crowding of the dentition. A lateral skull radiograph shows small hypophyseal fossa and small sinuses incompletely pneumatized.

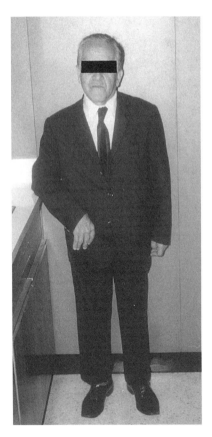

Figure 18–27
Pituitary dwarfism resulting from hypopituitarism. The individual is of small stature and proportionate body. Pituitary dwarfism must not be mistaken with achondroplastic dwarfism; in the latter, the extremities are short in comparison with the torso.

HYPERTHYROIDISM
(GRAVES' DISEASE, EXOPHTHALMIC GOITER, THYROTOXICOSIS)

In hyperthyroidism, there is excessive secretion of thyroxin by the thyroid gland. This excess thyroxin causes a generalized increase in the metabolic rate of all body tissues and results in tachycardia, nervous irritability, rapid pulse, fatigability, muscle weakness, heat intolerance and emaciation. There is protrusion of the eyeballs (exophthalmia) and enlargement of the thyroid gland (goiter). Radiographic findings include early eruption of permanent teeth after early exfoliation of deciduous teeth. Infants born to mothers with this condition may have several teeth at birth. Adults may show a generalized osteoporosis.

Most of the cases can eventually be controlled with treatment consisting either of administration of thyroid-suppressive drugs (or radioactive iodine) or of surgical removal of part of the thyroid gland. Use of certain drugs such as epinephrine and atropine is contraindicated because they may precipitate a potentially fatal complication called a thyroid storm.

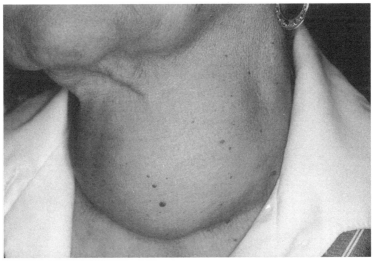

Figure 18–28
Hyperthyroidism. Enlargement of the thyroid gland in a patient with hyperthyroidism. (Courtesy Dr. Jim Cade).

HYPOTHYROIDISM

In hypothyroidism, there is deficient secretion of thyroxin by the thyroid gland. The congenital form is called cretinism and is marked by retarded physical, sexual and mental development. The individual will have short, fat, puffy features, sparse hair, delayed fusion of all bone epiphyses and fontanelles and an extremely large tongue causing separation of teeth. There is delayed eruption of teeth. The paranasal air sinuses show partial pneumatization.

The acquired form of hypothyroidism (in adults) is called myxedema and is marked by facial changes resulting in swollen lips and a thickened nose but no dental or skeletal changes (unlike cretinism). The symptoms in myxedema are lethargy, constipation, and cold intolerance. Treatment consists of exogenous replacement of thyroid hormone. The prognosis is good with treatment although finding the proper dosage of thyroxine often requires a trial and error approach. Without treatment, the disease is fatal.

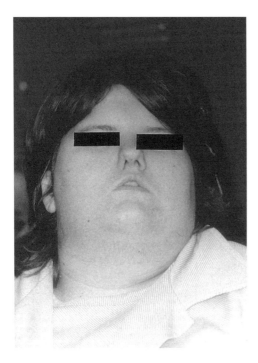

Figure 18–29
Cretinism resulting from hypothyroidism. The individual has short, fat, puffy features, and an extremely large tongue causing separation of teeth.

DIABETES MELLITUS

Diabetes mellitus results from an absence or decreased production of hormone insulin by the pancreas in response to elevated blood glucose. Predisposing factors include genetics, obesity, increasing age, pregnancy and stress. The condition is characterized by hyperglycemia, glycosuria, polyuria and polydipsia. Diabetes mellitus in itself does not cause periodontal disease; however, diabetic patients tend to have an increased incidence and severity of periodontal disease. There may be generalized loss of alveolar bone and a wide destruction of the lamina dura. Treatment includes a diet of low calories and low carbohydrates, hypoglycemic agents (which stimulate insulin production) and insulin injections (for severe cases). Death is usually due to myocardial infarction, renal failure, stroke or infection.

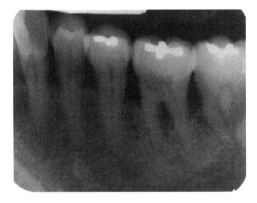

Figure 18–30
Diabetes mellitus. Uncontrolled diabetes mellitus shows loss of alveolar bone.

CUSHING'S SYNDROME

Cushing's syndrome is caused by hypersecretion of adrenal cortical hormones by the adrenal glands. Clinical signs and symptoms include central obesity, moon face (puffiness of face), buffalo hump (adipose tissue above the upper portion of the trunk), altered hair distribution (masculinizing effects in females and in male children), wasting of extremities, hypertension and a tendency to develop diabetes mellitus. On a radiograph, Cushing's syndrome exhibits generalized osteoporosis due to excess cortical activity. The osseous demineralization may lead to pathologic fractures. Patients undergoing exogenous steroid therapy should discontinue or reduce the dosage to cure the disease. When the cause is a cortisone-secreting tumor, it should be removed.

RICKETS AND OSTEOMALACIA

Rickets and osteomalacia result from a failure of new bone to properly calcify. The person has a nutritional deficiency of vitamin D combined with a lack of exposure to ultraviolet light. Rickets occurs in infants and children, whereas osteomalacia occurs in adults. In rickets, poor bone calcification results in bowing of long bones and increased widening of their epiphyses. Greenstick fractures may occur in these bones. Enamel hypoplasia is fairly common when rickets occurs before the age of 3 years. The teeth may show retarded apical closure and abnormally large pulp chambers. In osteomalacia the teeth are not affected because they are fully developed before the onset of the disease. Metastatic calcification occurs in many tissues (for example, renal stones).

In osteomalacia, the pain is localized in the bones; however, back pain is not as common as in osteoporosis. Spontaneous bone fractures may result. Radiographic changes are similar to those of osteoporosis and include generalized rarefaction and cortical thinning of bones. The lamina dura may be less prominent or completely absent. Treatment includes increased dosage of vitamin D and calcium supplements.

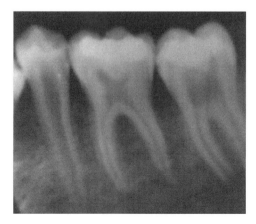

Figure 18–31
Rickets. Periapical radiograph shows rarefaction of bone and disappearance of lamina dura.

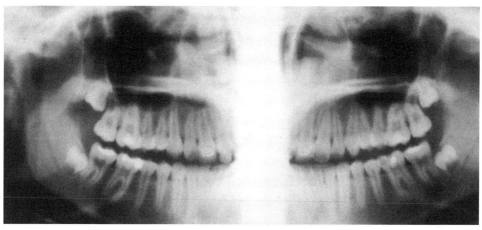

Figure 18–32
Osteomalacia. Panoramic radiograph shows osteoporosis of bone and disappearance of lamina dura.

HYPOPHOSPHATASIA

Hypophosphatasia is a hereditary disorder in which there is a deficiency of serum alkaline phosphatase. The clinical features include enlarged pulp chambers of deciduous teeth, alveolar bone loss with a predisposition for the anterior regions of the jaws, hypoplastic enamel and hypoplasia or aplasia of cementum over the root surface.

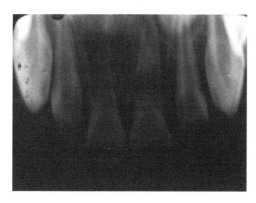

Figure 18–33
Hypophosphatasia. Teeth show thin enamel, thin root dentin, thin cementum and large pulp chambers.

401

OSTEOPOROSIS

Osteoporosis is a generalized rarefaction of bone without any change in size. The decreased mass is the result of increased porosity of compact bone and loss of trabeculae in cancellous bone. It is the most common form of metabolic bone disorder and is probably the most common cause of backache in elderly persons. Osteoporosis can occur from a number of causes; however, there is a greater tendency for it to occur in old age, postmenopausal women, Cushing's syndrome, hyperthyroidism, and patients receiving cortisone therapy. The bones are more prone to fracture. On a radiograph, osteoporosis is evident as a rarefaction of maxilla and mandible. The cortical borders of bone and anatomic cavities such as nasal fossa and maxillary sinus are thinner and less dense. Individual trabeculae are thin and fine. There is a reduction in the overall quantity of trabeculae in the cancellous bone. Treatment includes estrogen therapy, calcium supplements, protein, vitamin D, and fluoride.

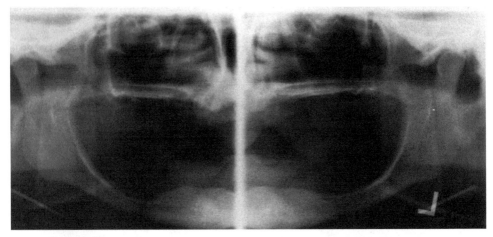

Figure 18–34

Osteoporosis. Panoramic radiograph of an elderly female shows a reduction in the overall quantity of trabeculae in the cancellous bone. The cortical bone is thin and less dense.

SCLERODERMA

Scleroderma is a systemic autoimmune disease of collagen. It is a generalized connective tissue disease that produces hardening and sclerosis of the skin. The age of onset of this rare disease is in the young to middle-aged adults. It is more common in females than in males (10:1). There is progressive fibrosis of all organs like the gastrointestinal tract, heart, lungs and kidneys which may result in serious complications and death. The facial skin and oral mucosa are rigid and the patient may be able to manage only limited mouth opening. There is marked thickening of the periodontal ligament spaces, especially around the posterior teeth. This periodontal ligament space thickening is about double the normal width. Another striking finding in 25 percent of scleroderma patients is the resorption of the mandibular condyles and coronoid processes. Treatment consists of immunosuppressants such as corticosteroids. The disease is debilitating but rarely fatal except over a long period of time. Death may occur due to progressive fibrosis of vital organs.

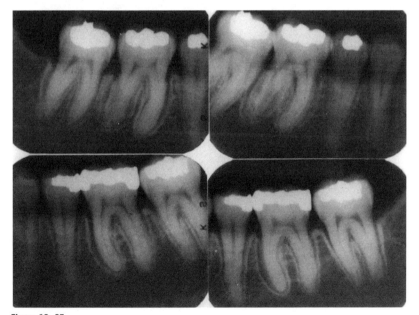

Figure 18–35

Scleroderma. Radiographs show generalized abnormal width of periodontal membrane space.

INFANTILE CORTICAL HYPEROSTOSIS (CAFFEY'S DISEASE)

Infantile cortical hyperostosis is a disease of unknown etiology. It is characterized by unusual cortical thickening of bones. The age of onset is usually in the first three months of life but may not be diagnosed until the age of 2 or 3 years. The mandible, clavicles, pelvis and extremities are most commonly affected. Soft tissue swellings occur over areas where bones will later be thickened. The symptoms are those of localized swelling, malocclusion with jaw involvement and increased alkaline phosphatase. The radiographic appearance is that of a laminated outer surface of bone caused by deposition of new bone under the periosteum. Most cases are self-limiting and regress without treatment within a few months or a few years. Rare cases produce permanent deformity.

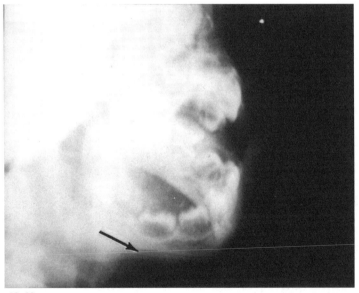

Figure 18–36
Infantile cortical hyperostosis. Lateral jaw radiograph shows the subperiosteal deposition of bone at the lower border of the mandible (arrow), giving it an onionskin appearance. (Courtesy Drs. Wuehrmann and Manson-Hing).

GENERALIZED RAREFACTIONS
Osteoporosis
Hyperparathyroidism
Osteomalacia
Hyperthyroidism
Cushing's syndrome
Prolonged cortisone therapy
Sickle cell anemia
Thalassemia
Leukemia

LOSS OF LAMINA DURA
Hyperparathyroidism
Paget's disease
Osteomalacia
Fibrous dysplasia
Cushing's syndrome

SERUM VALUES

Disorder	Calcium	Phosphorus	Alkaline Phosphatase
Osteoporosis	Normal	Normal	Normal
Primary Hyperparathyroidism	Increased	Decreased	Increased
Secondary Hyperparathyrodism	Normal to Decreased	Increased	Increased
Hypoparathyrodism	Decreased	Increased	Normal
Osteomalacia	Decreased	Decreased	Increased
Paget's disease	Normal	Normal	Increased
Multiple myeloma	Normal to Increased	Normal	Increased

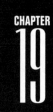

DIFFERENTIAL DIAGNOSIS OF COMMON LESIONS

1. PERIAPICAL RADIOLUCENCIES

Granuloma

Radicular cyst

Abscess

Apical scar

Surgical defect

Periodontal disease

Chronic suppurative osteomyelitis

Periapical cemental dysplasia (osteolytic stage)

Cementoblastoma (osteolytic stage)

Cementifying and ossifying fibromas (osteolytic stage)

Odontogenic and nonodontogenic cysts

Odontogenic and nonodontogenic benign tumors

Malignant tumors

2. PERIAPICAL RADIOPACITIES

Periapical cemental dysplasia (calcified stage)

Cementoblastoma (calcified stage)

Cementifying and ossifying fibromas (calcified stage)

Condensing osteitis

Osteosclerosis

Socket sclerosis

Florid osseous dysplasia (diffuse cementosis)

Tori

Hypercementosis

3. PERICORONAL RADIOLUCENCIES

Do not contain radiopacities:

   Follicular space

   Dentigerous cyst

   Mural ameloblastoma

   Odontogenic keratocyst

   Ameloblastoma

   Ameloblastic fibroma

May contain radiopacities:

   Ameloblastic fibro-odontoma

   Odontogenic adenomatoid tumor

   Calcifying epithelial odontogenic tumor (Pindborg tumor)

   Calcifying odontogenic cyst (Gorlin cyst)

4. SOLITARY CYSTLIKE RADIOLUCENCIES

Tooth follicle (early stage)

Large marrow space (wide inter-trabecular space)

Post extraction socket

Surgical defect

Odontogenic cysts:

Primordial

Lateral periodontal

Residual

Odontogenic keratocyst

Fissural cysts:

Incisive canal (nasopalatine)

Globulomaxillary

Median palatine

Median mandibular

False cysts:

Traumatic bone cyst

Stafne bone cavity

Odontogenic tumors:

Ameloblastoma

Odontogenic adenomatoid tumor

Calcified epithelial odontogenic tumor (Pindborg tumor)

Ameloblastic fibroma

Cementifying and ossifying fibromas (osteolytic stage)

Giant cell and nonodontogenic tumors:

    Central giant cell granuloma

    Giant cell lesion of hyperparathyroidism

    Non-odontogenic benign tumors

5. SOLITARY RADIOLUCENCIES WITH DIFFUSE IRREGULAR BORDERS

Chronic alveolar abscess

Chronic osteomyelitis

Osteoradionecrosis

Squamous cell carcinoma

Metastatic tumors to the jaws

Fibrous dysplasia (early stage)

Histiocytosis X

Osteosarcoma and chondrosarcoma

Ewing's sarcoma

Burkitt's lymphoma

6. MULTILOCULAR RADIOLUCENCIES

Cysts:

    Odontogenic keratocyst (basal cell nevus syndrome)

    Aneurysmal bone cyst

Tumors:

    Ameloblastoma

    Odontogenic myxoma

    Central hemangioma of bone

    Metastatic tumors to the jaws

Others:

    Cherubism

    Central giant cell granuloma

    Giant cell lesion of hyperparathyroidism

7. SOLITARY RADIOPACITIES

Exostoses and tori

Osteoma

Retained root

Osteosclerosis

Socket sclerosis

Complex composite odontoma

Compound composite odontoma

Calcifications in soft tissue

Foreign objects in the jaws

Fibrous dysplasia

Garré's osteomyelitis

8. MIXED RADIOLUCENT—RADIOPAQUE LESIONS

Condensing osteitis

Osteomyelitis:

Chronic suppurative osteomyelitis

Tuberculous osteomyelitis

Syphilitic osteomyelitis

Actinomycotic osteomyelitis

Osteoradionecrosis

Cementomas (intermediate and calcified stages):

Periapical cemental dysplasia

Cementifying and ossifying fibroma

Cementoblastoma

Florid osseous dysplasia (diffuse cementosis)

Others:

Fibrous dysplasia

Paget's disease

Osteosarcoma

Chondrosarcoma

Osteoblastic metastatic carcinoma

Pericoronal mixed lesions:

Ameloblastic fibro-odontoma

Odontogenic adenomatoid tumor

Calcifying epithelial odontogenic tumor (Pindborg tumor)

Calcifying odontogenic cyst (Gorlin cyst)

9. GENERALIZED RADIOPACITIES

Florid osseous dysplasia (diffuse cementosis)

Paget's disease

Osteopetrosis

Gardner's syndrome

Infantile cortical hyperostosis

INDEX

A

Abrasion 200, 202

Abscess 110–113, 407, 410

Achondroplasia 377–378

Acromegaly 394–395

Actinomycotic osteomyelitis 275, 412

Adenoameloblastoma 284–286, 264, 408, 409, 412

Adenomatoid odontogenic tumor 284–286, 264, 408, 409, 412

Albers–Schönberg disease 370, 371, 358, 413

Albright's syndrome 320–323

Ameloblastic fibroma 288–290, 361, 408, 409

Ameloblastic fibro-odontoma 291–293, 408, 412

Ameloblastic odontoma 291

Ameloblastoma 280–284, 361, 408, 409, 411

Ameloblastoma, mural 235, 236, 264, 265, 280, 408

Amelogenesis imperfecta 209, 210, 196, 197, 207

Amputation neuroma 315–317

Aneurysmal bone cyst 256, 257, 410

Angulation effects on
    caries 75–90
    crestal bone height 96, 99
    foreshortening and elongation 139, 140

Ankylosed teeth 205, 206

Anodontia 181–183 ,366, 367

Anomalies 169–216
    abration 200, 202

amelogenesis imperfecta 209, 210, 196, 197, 207
ankylosed teeth 205, 206
anodontia 181–183, 366, 367
attrition 200–202
concrescence 192, 193
dens in dente 193–195
dens evaginatus 195
dentinal dysplasia 212, 213
dentinogenesis imperfecta 211, 212, 207, 369
dilaceration 197, 198
enamel pearl 199, 200
enameloma 199, 200
erosion 201
fusion 189–191
gemination 191, 192
hypercementosis 198, 135, 388–390, 408
hypodontia 181–183, 366, 367
hypoplasia 206–208, 209, 210
idiopathic resorption 174, 175
impacted teeth 203, 204
macrodontia 187, 188
mesiodens 186, 187
microdontia 188, 189
odontodysplasia 214–216
odontogenesis imperfecta 214–216
pathologic resorption 176–178
physiologic resorption 172, 173
pulp calcifications 178–181
pulpal obliteration 179–181
pulp stones 179
reparative dentin 179, 180
resorption 171–178
secondary dentin 179, 180

submerged teeth 203
supernumerary teeth 183–186
talon cusp 196
taurodontism 196, 197
tooth resorption 171–178
transposed teeth 204, 205
Turner's hypoplasia 208, 207

Antral retention cyst 258, 259, 351

Antrolith 224, 352, 353

Apical abscess 110–113, 407

Apical cementoma 124–127, 407, 408, 412

Apical cyst 110–113, 237, 238, 407

Apical granuloma 110–113, 407

Apical lesions
apical abscess 110–113, 407, 410
apical cyst 110–113, 237, 238, 407
apical periodontitis 105–108
apical scar 113, 114, 407
cementifying fibroma 125, 128 129, 300–303, 362, 407–409, 412
cementoblastoma, benign 125, 127, 128, 303, 304, 407, 408, 412
cementomas 124–129, 300–304, 407, 408, 412
cementosis, diffuse 130–132, 408, 412, 413
chronic diffuse sclerosing osteomyelitis 130–132, 408, 412, 413
condensing osteitis 117, 118, 408, 412

differential diagnosis 135, 407, 408

florid osseous dysplasia 130–132, 408, 412, 413

focal sclerosing osteomyelitis 117, 118, 408, 412

gigantiform cementoma 130 132, 408, 412, 413

granuloma 110–113, 407

hypercementosis 198, 135, 388, 390, 408

medullary spaces 133

osteosclerosis 119–123, 408, 411

periapical cemental dysplasia 124–127, 407, 408, 412

periapical granuloma 110–113, 407

periapical radiolucencies 135, 407

periapical radiopacities 135, 408

periodontal disease 116, 91–102, 407

periodontal space widening 105–108

radicular cyst 110–113, 237, 238, 407

socket sclerosis 119, 121, 122, 408, 411

surgical defect 114, 115, 407, 409

tori 133, 134, 305, 306

Apical periodontitis 105–108

Apical scar 113, 114, 407

Arteries, calcification of 223

Arteriovenous fistula 312

Artifacts 137–153

Attrition 200–202

B

Basal cell nevus syndrome 242–245, 410

Beam angulation effects on
caries 86–90
crestal bone height 96–99
foreshortening and elongation 139, 140

Benign cementoblastoma 125, 127, 128, 303, 304, 407, 408, 412

Bifid ribs basal cell nevus syndrome 242–244, 410

Brittle bones disease 368, 369

Brown tumors 391, 393

Buccal caries 79, 80

Burkitt's lymphoma 341

Burnout
cervical 83–85, 82
peripheral 83, 106

C

Caffey's disease 404

Calcification of arteries 223

Calcifications, pulpal 178–181

Calcified lymph node 272, 220, 221

Calcified stylohyoid ligament and Eagle's syndrome 226–228

Calcified thyroid cartilage 228, 229

Calcifying epithelial odontogenic cyst 246, 247, 408, 412

Calcifying epithelial odontogenic tumor 287, 288, 408, 409, 412

Calcinosis cutis 225

Calculus 92, 93

Carcinoma, squamous cell 327–330, 363, 410

Carcinoma, metastatic 330–332, 410

Caries 75–90
    beam angulation effects on, 86–90
    cemental 81
    facial and lingual 79, 80
    proximal caries 77, 78
    occlusal 75–77
    recurrent 82;
    root 81

Cemental caries 81

Cemental dysplasia 124–127, 407, 408, 412

Cementifying fibroma 125, 128, 129, 300–303, 362, 407–409, 412

Cementoblastoma, 125, 127, 128, 303, 304, 407, 408, 412

Cementomas,

cementifying fibroma 125, 128, 129, 300–303, 362, 407–409, 412

cementoblastoma 125, 127, 128, 303, 304, 407, 408, 412

cemento-ossifying fibroma 125, 128, 129, 300–303, 362, 407–409, 412

chronic sclerosing cementosis 130–132, 408, 412, 413

diffuse cementosis 130–132, 408, 412, 413

diffuse sclerosing osteomyelitis 130–132, 408, 412, 413

gigantiform cementoma 130–132, 408, 412, 413

multiple enostoses 130–132, 408, 412, 413

ossifying fibroma 125 ,128, 129, 300–303, 362, 407–409, 412

periapical cemental dysplasia 124–127, 407, 408, 412

periapical cementoma 124–127, 407, 408, 412

Cementosis, diffuse 130–132, 408, 412, 413

Cemento-ossifying fibroma 125, 128, 129, 300–303, 362, 407–409, 412

Central giant cell granuloma 318–320, 358, 391, 393, 410, 411

Central hemangioma 310–312, 411

Cervical burnout 83–85, 82

Cherubism 367, 368, 411

Chondroma 317

Chondrosarcoma 333, 410, 412

Chronic diffuse sclerosing osteomyelitis 130 –132, 408, 412, 413

Chronic sclerosing cementosis 130–132, 408, 412, 413

Chronic suppurative osteomyelitis 267–269, 407, 410, 412

Clefts of the jaw bones 378, 379, 183

Cleidocranial dysostosis 371–373, 183, 184, 207

Coin test 152

Complex composite odontoma 294–297, 411

Compound composite odontoma 293–295, 411

Concrescence 192, 193

Condensing osteitis 117, 118, 408, 412

Cone-cut 142, 143

Cooley's anemia 382 –384

Cotton-wool appearance 388–390

Craniofacial dysostosis 373–375

Crouzon's disease 373–375

Cushing's syndrome 399, 405

Cysticercosis 230

Cysts

aneurysmal bone 256, 257, 410

antral retention 258, 259, 351

apical 110–113, 237, 238, 407

calcifying odontogenic 246, 247, 408, 412

definition of 232

dental 110–113, 237, 238, 407

dentigerous 235–237, 408

developmental defect 260–262, 409

differential diagnosis of odontogenic cysts 264, 265

differential diagnosis of radiolucencies around tooth crowns 264, 265, 408

extravasation bone 254–256, 409

facial or fissural 232, 248–253, 409

follicular 235 –237, 408

globulomaxillary 248, 409

Gorlin 246, 247, 408, 412

hemorrhagic 254–256, 409

idiopathic bone 254–256, 409

incisive canal 250 –252, 409

infected 110–113, 237, 238, 407

inflammatory 110–113, 237, 238, 407

intraosseous hematoma 254–256, 409

keratocyst 241–243, 408–410

latent bone 260–262, 409

lateral periodontal 239, 409

lingual cortical defect of mandible 260–262, 409

median alveolar 249, 409

median mandibular 249, 409

median palatal 252, 409

mucoid retention 258, 259, 351

mucous retention 258, 259, 351

nasoalveolar 253

nasolabial 253

nasopalatine canal 250–252, 409

nonodontogenic 232, 248–262

odontogenic 232, 233–247

odontogenic keratocyst 241–243, 408–410

periapical 110–113, 237, 238, 407

periodontal 110–113, 237, 238, 409

primordial 235–237, 409

radicular 110–113, 237, 238, 407

radiolucencies misdiagnosed as 262, 263

residual 240, 241, 409

simple bone 254–256, 409

sinus mucocele 258, 259, 351

solitary bone 254–256, 409

Stafne bone 260–262, 409

static bone 260–262, 409

traumatic bone 254–256, 409

Cysts in maxillary sinus 351, 357, 358, 258, 259

D

Dens in dente 193–195

Dens evaginatus 195

Dens invaginatus 193–195

Density of films 138

Dental abscess 110–113, 407, 410

Dental cyst 110–113, 237, 238, 407

Denticles 179

Dentigerous cyst 235–237, 408

Dentin, reparative 179, 180

Dentin, secondary 179, 180

Dentinal dysplasia 212, 213

Dentinogenesis imperfecta 211, 212, 207, 369

Dentoalveolar abscess 110–113, 407, 410

Developmental defect cyst 260–262, 409

Diabetes mellitus 101, 399

Differential diagnosis of
generalized radiopacities 413
mixed radiolucent-radiopaque lesions 412
multilocular radiolucencies 410, 411
odontogenic cysts 264
periapical radiolucencies 135, 407
periapical radiopacities 135, 408
pericoronal radiolucencies 264, 265, 408

pericoronal radiolucency around crown of anterior tooth 264, 408

pericoronal radiolucency around crown of posterior tooth 265, 408

solitary cystlike radiolucencies 409, 410

solitary radiolucencies with diffuse irregular borders 410

solitary radiopacities 411

Diffuse cementosis 130–132, 408, 412, 413

Diffuse sclerosing osteomyelitis, chronic 130–132, 408, 412, 413

Dilaceration 197, 198

Dilated composite odontoma 193–195

Distodens 183, 185

Distomolar 183, 185

Dwarfism
achondroplastic 377, 378
pituitary 396

E

Eagle's syndrome 226–228

Ectodermal Dysplasia 366, 367, 181, 182

Elongation 139, 140

Enamel hypocalcification 209, 210

Enamel hypoplasia 209, 210

Enamel pearl 199, 200

Enameloma 199, 200

Enostoses 119, 120, 130–132

Eosinophilic granuloma 324, 325

Epidermolysis bullosa dystrophica 207

Erosion 201

Errors
See Technique Errors and Artifacts 137–153

Erythroblastic anemia 382–384

Ewing's sarcoma 334, 410

Exophthalmic goiter 397

Exostoses and tori 305–307, 5, 13, 24, 31, 32, 133, 134, 411

Extravasation bone cyst 254–256, 409

F

Facial caries 79, 80

Facial cleft cysts 232, 248–253, 409

Familial intraosseous swellings of jaws 367, 368, 411

Familial multilocular cystic disease of jaws 367, 368, 411

Fibroma, odontogenic 300

Fibrosarcoma 334

Fibrous dysplasia 320–323, 359, 405, 410–412

Fissural cysts 232, 248–253, 409

Floating in air teeth 323, 324, 328

Florid osseous dysplasia 130–132, 408, 412, 413

Fluorosis, endemic 207

Focal sclerosing osteomyelitis 117, 118, 408, 412

Fogged film 151

Follicular cyst 235–237, 408

Foreign bodies 155–167

Foreshortening 139, 140

Fragilitas ossium 368, 369, 207, 211

Fusion 189–191

G

Gardner's syndrome 386, 387, 183, 413

Garré's osteomyelitis 270, 271, 411

Gemination 191, 192

Genetic diseases
    achondroplasia 377, 378
    cherubism 367, 368, 411
    cleft of the lip and palate 378, 379
    cleidocranial dysostosis 371–373, 183, 184
    craniofacial dysostosis 373–375
    Crouzon's syndrome 373–375
    ectodermal dysplasia 366, 367, 181, 182
    Gardner's syndrome 386, 387, 183, 413
    hemifacial hypertrophy 385, 386
    hemifacial hypoplasia 384, 385
    mandibulofacial dysostosis 375, 376
    maxillary sinus affected 358, 359
    osteogenesis imperfecta 368, 369, 207, 211
    osteopetrosis 370, 371, 358, 413
    Pierre Robin syndrome 379, 380
    sickle cell anemia 380–382
    thalassemia 382–384
    Treacher Collins syndrome 375, 376

Ghost teeth 214–216

Giant cell granuloma, central 318–320, 358, 391, 410, 411

Giant cell lesion of hyperparathyroidism 391–393, 410, 411

Gigantiform cementomas 130–132, 408, 412, 413

Gigantism 394

Globulomaxillary cyst 248, 409

Gorlin cyst 246, 247, 408, 412

Granuloma, periapical 110–113, 407

Graves' disease 397

Ground glass appearance 320–322, 391, 392

H

Hair-on-end appearance 381–383

Hamartoma
    complex 294–298
    compound 293–295

Hand-Schüller-Christian disease 323, 324, 326

Hemangioma, central 310–312, 222, 411

Hemifacial hypertrophy 385, 386

Hemifacial hypoplasia 384, 385

Hemorrhagic cyst 254–256, 409

Hereditary fibrous dysplasia 367, 368

Hereditary opalescent dentin 211, 212

Herringbone effect 145

Histiocytosis X 323–326, 102, 410

Honeycomb effect 145

Hypercementosis 198, 135, 388–390, 408

Hyperostosis 123

Hyperparathyroidism 391–393, 405, 410, 411

Hyperpituitarism 394, 395

Hyperthyroidism 397, 405

Hypocalcification, enamel 209

Hypodontia 181–183, 366, 367

Hypoparathyroidism 393, 405

Hypophosphatasia 401

Hypopituitarism 396

Hypoplasia 207–210

Hypoplasia, Turner's 207, 208

Hypothyroidism 398

I

Idiopathic bone cyst 254–256, 409

Idiopathic resorption 174, 175

Impacted teeth 203, 204

Incisive canal cyst 250–252, 409

Infantile cortical hyperostosis 404, 413

Infected cyst 110–113, 237, 238, 407

Inflammatory cyst 110–113, 237, 238 ,407

Interproximal caries 77–79

Intraosseous hematoma 254–256, 409

Irradiation effects on developing teeth 276, 278

J

Juvenile periodontitis 100, 101

K

Keratinizing and calcifying cyst 246, 247, 408, 412

Keratocyst, odontogenic 241–243, 408–410

Klinefelter's syndrome 196, 197

L

Lamina dura 92, 93

Langerhans' cell granulomatosis 323–326

Latent bone cyst 260–262, 409

Lateral periodontal cyst 239, 409

Letterer-Siwe disease 323, 324

Leukemia 336, 337, 405

Lingual caries 79, 80

Lingual cortical defect of mandible 260–262

Lingual tori 133–135, 305–307, 408, 411

Lobstein's disease 368, 369, 207, 211

Lymph node calcification 272, 220, 221

Lymphomas, malignant 340

Lymphoma, Burkitt's 341, 410

M

Macrodontia 187, 188

Malignant lymphomas 340

Malignant tumors of the jaws
  Burkitt's lymphoma 341, 410
  leukemia 336, 337
  malignant lymphomas 340
  metastatic carcinoma 330–332, 410
  multiple myeloma 337–340
  sarcomas 332–336, 410, 412
  squamous cell carcinoma 327–330, 410

Mandible developmental bone defect 260–262, 409

Mandibular tori 305–307, 133–135, 408, 411

Mandibulofacial dysostosis 375–376

Marble bone disease 370, 371, 358, 413

Maxillary sinus 343–364

ameloblastic fibro-odontoma 361

ameloblastoma 361

antral retention cyst 258, 259, 351

antrolith 224, 352, 353

carcinoma, squamous cell 363

cementifying fibroma 362

cysts, odontogenic and nonodontogenic 357, 358

fibrous dysplasia 359

foreign objects 352–354

genetic, metabolic and tumor-like diseases 358, 359

hyperplastic mucosa 347, 348

mucous retention cyst 258, 259, 351

myxoma, odontogenic 362

normal, variations of 344, 345

odontoma 360

oro-antral fistula 355, 356

ossifying fibroma 362

osteoma 360

osteopetrosis 358

osteosarcoma 364

Paget's disease 359

pneumatization 345

sinusitis 346–350

tumors 360–364

Maxillary sinusitis 346 –350

Median alveolar cyst 249

Median mandibular cyst 249, 409

Median palatal cyst 252, 409

Mediterranean anemia 382–384

Medullary spaces 133

Megadontia 187, 188

Mesiodens 186, 187

Metabolic diseases
Cushing's syndrome 399, 405
diabetes mellitus 101, 399
hyperparathyroidism 391–393, 405, 410, 411
hyperpituitarism 394, 395
hyperthyroidism 397, 405
hypoparathyroidism 393, 405
hypophosphatasia 401
hypopituitarism 396
hypothyroidism 398
infantile cortical hyperostosis 404, 413
maxillary sinus affected 358, 359
osteomalacia 400, 401, 405
osteoporosis 402, 405
Paget's disease 387–390, 359, 405, 413
rickets 400
scleroderma 403

Metastatic carcinoma 330–332, 410

Microdontia 188, 189

Miliary osteomas of skin 225

Mucocele in sinus 258, 259, 351

Mucoid retention cyst in maxillary sinus 258, 259, 351

Mucous retention cyst in maxillary sinus 258, 259, 351

Multiple enostoses 130–132, 408, 412, 413

Multiple miliary osteomas of skin 225

Multiple myeloma 337–340, 405

Mural ameloblastoma 235, 236, 264, 265, 280, 408

Myositis ossificans 229

Myxofibroma 298, 299, 362, 411

Myxoma, odontogenic 298, 299, 362, 411

N

Nasoalveolar cyst 253

Nasolabial cyst 253

Nasopalatine canal cyst 250–252, 409

Neurilemmoma 313, 314

Neurofibroma 313–315

Neurogenic tumors 313–317

Neuroma
    amputation 315, 316
    traumatic 315, 316

Nonodontogenic benign tumors of the jaws
    arteriovenous fistula 312
    chondroma 317

exostoses and tori 305–307, 133–135, 408, 411

fibrous dysplasia 320–323, 359, 405, 410–412

giant cell granuloma, central 318–320, 358, 391, 393, 410, 411

hemangioma, central 310–312, 222, 411

histiocytosis X 323–326, 102, 410

neurogenic tumors (neurilemmoma, neurofibroma) 313–317

osteoid osteoma 309, 310

osteoma 307–309, 411

traumatic neuroma 315–317

Nonodontogenic cysts
    in jaws. See Cysts
    in maxillary sinus 357, 358

O

Occlusal caries 75–77

Odontodysplasia 214–216

Odontogenesis imperfecta 214–216

Odontogenic adenomatoid tumor 284–286, 264, 408, 409, 412

Odontogenic cysts
    in jaws. See Cysts
    in maxillary sinus 357, 358, 351

Odontogenic fibroma 300

Odontogenic keratocyst 241–243, 408–410

Odontogenic myxoma (myxofibroma) 298, 299, 362, 411

Odontogenic tumors
  adenomatoid odontogenic tumor 284–286, 264, 408, 409, 412
  ameloblastic fibroma 288–290, 361, 408, 409
  ameloblastic fibro-odontoma 291–293, 408, 412
  ameloblastic odontoma 291
  ameloblastoma 280–284, 361, 408, 409, 411
  calcifying epithelial tumor 287, 288, 408, 409, 412
  cementifying fibroma 125, 128, 129, 300–303, 362, 407–409, 412
  cemento-ossifying fibroma 125, 128, 129, 300–303, 362, 407–409, 412
  cementoblastoma 125, 127, 128, 303, 304, 407, 408, 412
  complex composite odontoma 294–297, 411
  compound composite odontoma 293–295, 411
  hamatoma 293–298, 411
  myxofibroma 298, 299, 362, 411
  odontogenic adenomatoid tumor 284–286, 264, 408, 409, 412
  odontogenic fibroma 300
  odontogenic myxoma 298, 299, 362, 411
  odontoma 293–295, 411

  ossifying fibroma 125, 128, 129, 300–303, 362, 407–409, 412
  Pindborg tumor 287, 288, 408, 409, 412

Odontoma
  complex 294–297, 411
  compound 293–295, 411

Oligodontia 181

Onion-skin appearance 270–271,

Opalescent dentin, hereditary 211, 212

Oro-antral fistula 355, 356

Ossifying fibroma 125, 128, 129, 300–303, 362, 407–409, 412

Osteitis deformans 387–390, 359, 412, 413

Osteogenesis imperfecta 368, 369, 207, 211

Osteogenic sarcoma 333, 335, 336, 364, 410, 412

Osteoid osteoma 309, 310

Osteoma 307–309, 360, 411

Osteoma cutis 225

Osteomas of skin 225

Osteomalacia 400, 401 405

Osteomyelitis
  actinomycotic 275, 412
  chronic diffuse sclerosing 130–132, 408, 412, 413
  focal sclerosing 117, 118

Garré's 270, 271, 411

osteoradionecrosis 276–278, 410, 412

periostitis ossificans 270, 271, 411

suppurative 267–269, 407, 410, 412

syphilitic 273, 274, 412

tuberculous 271, 272, 412

Osteopetrosis 370, 371, 358, 413

Osteoporosis 402, 405

Osteoporotic bone marrow defect 262, 32, 133

Osteoradionecrosis 276–278, 410, 412

Osteosarcoma 333, 335, 336, 364, 410, 412

Osteosclerosis 119–123, 408, 411

P

Paget's disease 387–390, 359, 412, 413

Palatal caries 79, 80

Panoramic radiography
anatomy 41–50
patient positioning errors 51–56

Papillon-Lefèvre syndrome 100

Paramolar 183, 185

Pathologic resorption 176, 177

Peg laterals 188, 189

Periapical cemental dysplasia 124–127, 407, 408, 412

Periapical cementoma 124–127, 407, 408, 412

Periapical cyst 110–113, 237, 238, 407

Periapical granuloma 110–113, 407

Periapical lesions
see apical lesions

Periapical radiolucencies, differential diagnosis 135, 407

Periapical radiopacities, differential diagnosis 135, 408

Pericoronal radiolucencies, differential diagnosis 264, 265, 408

Peridens 183

Periodontal cyst 110–113, 237, 238, 409

Periodontal disease 91–102, 116

Periodontal space widening 105–108, 94

Periodontitis, juvenile 100, 101

Periodontosis, juvenile 100, 101

Periostitis ossificans 270, 271, 411

Peripheral burnout 83, 106

Phlebolith 222

Physiologic resorption 172, 173

Pierre Robin syndrome 379, 380

Pindborg tumor 287, 288, 408, 409, 412

Primordial cyst 235–237, 409

Proximal caries 77, 78

Pulp calcifications 178–181

Pulpal obliteration 179, 180

Pulp stones 178, 179

R

Radicular cyst 110–113, 237, 238, 407

Recurrent caries 82

Reparative dentin 179–180

Residual cyst 240, 241, 409

Resorption
    idiopathic 174, 175
    pathologic 176–178
    physiologic 172–173

Reticulation 148

Reticuloendotheliosis 323

Rickets 400

Root caries 81

S

Sarcoma
    chondrosarcoma 333, 410, 412
    Ewing's sarcoma 334, 410
    fibrosarcoma 334
    osteosarcoma 333, 335, 336, 410, 412

Scar
    apical 113, 114, 407
    surgical 114, 115, 407, 409

Schwannoma 313, 314

Scleroderma 403, 102

Sclerosing cementosis 130–132, 408, 412, 413

Sclerosing osteomyelitis, chronic diffuse 130–132, 408, 412, 413

Secondary dentin 179, 180

Sequestrum 268 ,269, 272, 276, 277

Sialolith 217–220

Sickle cell anemia 380–382, 404

Simple bone cyst 254–256, 409

Sinus mucocele 258, 259, 351

Sinusitis, maxillary 346–350

Soap bubble appearance 280

Socket sclerosis 119, 121, 122, 408, 411

Solitary bone cyst 254–256, 409

Squamous cell carcinoma 327–330, 363, 410

Stafne bone cavity 260–262, 409

Static bone cavity 260–262, 409

Static electricity 152, 153

Stepladder appearance 181, 182

Stylohyoid ligament, calcification 226–228

Submerged teeth 203

Supernumerary teeth 183–186, 371–373, 379, 386

Supplemental teeth 183

Suppurative osteomyelitis 267–269, 407, 410, 412

Surgical defect 114, 115, 407, 409

Synodontia 189–191

Syphilitic
    osteomyelitis 273, 274
    hypoplasia, prenatal or congenital 207

T

Talon cusp 196

Taurodontism 196, 197

Technique errors and artifacts 137–153

Thalassemia 382–384, 405

Thyroid cartilage, calcification 228, 229

Thyrotoxicosis 397

Tooth resorption; see resorption

Torus
    mandibularis 305–307, 133–135, 408, 411
    palatinus 305–307, 133–135, 408, 411

Transposed teeth 204, 205

Traumatic bone cyst 254–256, 409

Traumatic neuroma 315, 316

Treacher Collins syndrome 375, 376

Tricho-dento-osseous syndrome 196, 197

Tuberculous osteomyelitis 271, 272